Type 2 Diabetes Cookbook FOR BEGINNERS

—— 600 ——

Easy and Type 2 Diabetes Friendly Recipes for Beginners On a Budget

Josephine Durrett

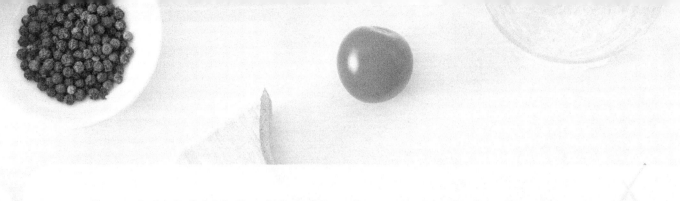

Copyright© 2022 By Josephine Durrett All Rights Reserved

This book is copyright protected. It is only for personal use. You cannot amend, distribute, sell, use, quote or paraphrase any part of the content within this book, without the consent of the author or publisher.

Under no circumstances will any blame or legal responsibility be held against the publisher, or author, for any damages, reparation, or monetary loss due to the information contained within this book, either directly or indirectly.

Disclaimer Notice:

Please note the information contained within this document is for educational and entertainment purposes only. All effort has been executed to present accurate, up to date, reliable, complete information. No warranties of any kind are declared or implied. Readers acknowledge that the author is not engaged in the rendering of legal, financial, medical or professional advice. The content within this book has been derived from various sources. Please consult a licensed professional before attempting any techniques outlined in this book.

By reading this document, the reader agrees that under no circumstances is the author responsible for any losses, direct or indirect, that are incurred as a result of the use of the information contained within this document, including, but not limited to, errors, omissions, or inaccuracies.

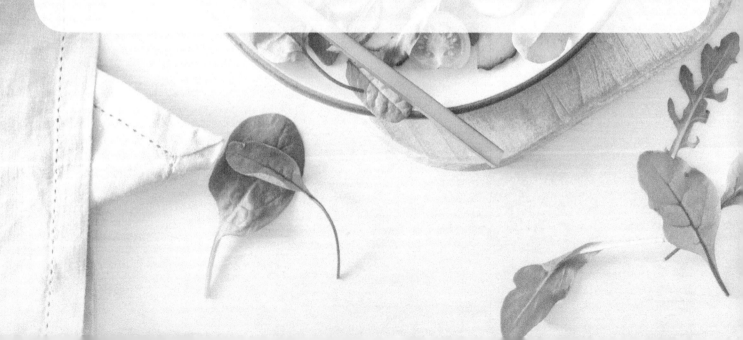

CONTENT

Introduction		1
Chapter 1	Breakfasts	8
Chapter 2	Vegetables and Sides	19
Chapter 3	Staples, Sauces, Dips, and Dressings	29
Chapter 4	Beef, Pork, and Lamb	34
Chapter 5	Poultry	47
Chapter 6	Fish and Seafood	60
Chapter 7	Salads	70
Chapter 8	Desserts	80
Chapter 9	Stews and Soups	89
Appendix 1	Measurement Conversion Chart	100
Appendix 2	The Dirty Dozen and Clean Fifteen	101
Appendix 3	Recipes Index	102

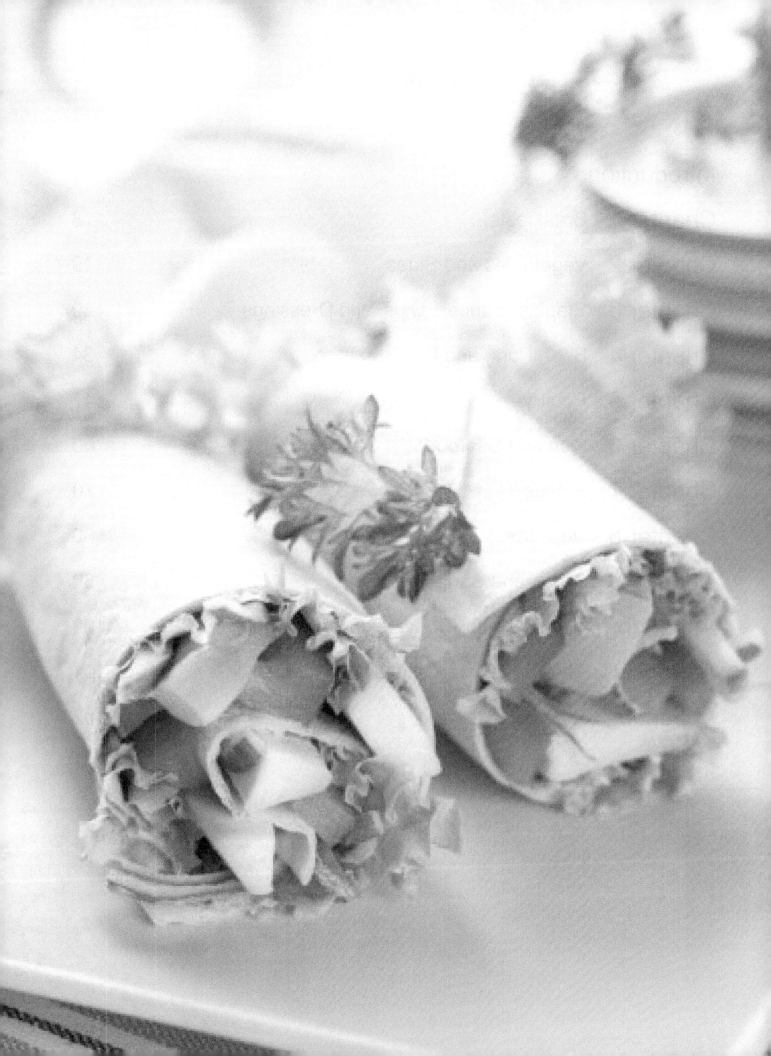

INTRODUCTION

A year ago, I was diagnosed with Type 2 diabetes. I was overweight and a total sugar and carb addict. The doctor told me that I would need to be on medication and have to live with this disease for the rest of my life. I watched my father suffer and die from diabetes. I saw him inject insulin every day and I don't want to end up like him. I was worried and became obsessed with finding a cure. So I did my research. I saw many videos and read many books on diabetes, but none of these videos and books gave a simple and straightforward approach to managing diabetes. Due to the lack of simple materials in managing the situation, I did a tremendous amount of research and a realized food management, healthy living, and exercise are the most important factors in type 2 diabetics management.

My simple Type 2 diabetes management method gave me hope. At that point, I committed myself to a strict diet. I did this diet as if my life depended on it. I ate fewer carbohydrates a day and avoided sugar. I checked my blood sugar level at least six times a day to get a complete picture of what everything did to my blood glucose levels. After six weeks, my blood sugar was perfect for a non-diabetic. No medicine. Just diet and exercise. It has now been about ten months. I now do a moderate carb and fat diet. Very little red meat. Fish, chicken, lots of veggies and salads with oil and vinegar, cheeses, and whole grain bread. During winter and I eat pasta, some pizza, and plenty fruit. No sugars. On rare occasions, I eat chocolate. I check my blood glucose levels every morning before breakfast. My blood glucose level never exceeds 5.6 (100). It usually ranges from 4.3 to 5.2, even if I have pasta or pizza at dinner. I do my best to live with as little stress as possible and have a quality sleep.

By following this lifestyle that was extensively built on healthy diet management, I was able to reverse diabetes. I am not alone in this. There are thousands of people who have similar stories. Some people sincerely believe that Type 2 diabetes is an irreversible and progressive disease. They are only repeating what they have been told by the pharmaceutical and medical industries who have a financial interest in not curing diabetes. I am inspired to write this book because of you. The 200 recipes, 21-day meal plan in this cookbook are new alternatives that offer hope and have greatly helped me manage my diabetes, and I believe it will greatly help you too.

Some people are born with diabetes; however, millions of people are diagnosed with Type 2 diabetes every year—otherwise called adult-onset diabetes. Upon diagnosis, if you're like me, you are likely to be upset, confused, and unsure of where to turn. This introductory cookbook is designed to help newly diagnosed Type 2 diabetics patients ease into a new diet and way of living. Type 2 Diabetes Cookbook for Beginners is a must to help you learn. You'll find over 200 helpful recipes as well as advice and general information for living with diabetes. This book is loaded with 21-days delectable meal plan, so in case you're worried you'll have to live the rest of your life eating tasteless food, don't be.

When you're diagnosed with Type 2 diabetes, blood glucose levels are a constant concern. However, with the proper eating routine, you wouldn't have to worry. We all love tasty food; good meatloaf, creamy mac, and cheese or wholesome spaghetti with meatballs. Unfortunately, many people believe that a diabetes diagnosis means they cannot enjoy these tasty foods. In reality, it only takes some extra care with ingredients and a couple of minor adjustments to recipes to update these tasty foods for a low-glycemic diet. Like every great cookbook, Type 2 Diabetes Cookbook for Beginners is sprinkled with convenient kitchen tips and time-efficient guidance, making it an excellent choice for someone trying to eat more healthily without forfeiting their favorite foods.

This extensive cookbook of diabetes-friendly recipes is designed with love to be perfectly portioned for people with Type 2 diabetes. Regardless of whether you're trying to forestall or control diabetes, your nutritional requirements are almost the same as everyone's. However, you do have to focus on some diet choices, especially carbohydrates. While exercising and living healthy can help, the most important thing you can do is eat healthy. Eating healthy can help you lose a large percentage of your total weight, lower blood pressure, blood sugar, and cholesterol levels. Eating healthier can likewise have a significant impact on mood, energy, and sense of well-being.

Getting diagnosed with diabetes can be terrifying, particularly if you have no idea of the next steps to take. You might start to ask yourself, "Should I be on medicine and supplements? Should I enroll in an exercise program? Should I do this? Should I do that?" These are the thoughts that will run through your mind, and these processes can be overwhelming. However, the most important decision that I made was changing my diet plan. Food is a fundamental part of our survival, and we love to eat. For an individual with diabetes, this doesn't need to change. You don't need to forfeit food for diabetes.

Notwithstanding, exposing yourself to new recipes and meal ideas is never a bad thing. You should simply change your prediabetes favorites into healthier food alternatives. The flavor shouldn't be an issue because there are several ways you can augment your meals to keep them delightful yet healthier. This is where the Type 2 Diabetes Cookbook for Beginners can help. This book will change your eating habits for the better. This cookbook has advice and recipes for all lifestyles, regardless of whether you are battling with portion control or eating out or simply don't have time to prepare a meal every night.

It's significant for individuals with diabetes to monitor their diets intently, as the disease incredibly increases one's risk of heart attack or stroke. This comprehensive cookbook includes snacks and dessert and doesn't forfeit taste for healthy dieting. Sometimes, we all crave for snacks, right? For most people, meal planning is challenging and tends to be much more challenging for diabetic patients. This cookbook recommends people with diabetes fill their dinner plates with veggies, protein, starch, or grain. All the recipes in the book follow standard basic portioning, allowing you to mix different components of various diet as you wish. This straightforward approach makes the process of building healthy and delicious meals simpler.

The overall objective of this book is to give hope to Type 2 diabetes patients by helping them manage their condition through the provision of essential information, fundamental skills, resources, and support expected to achieve optimal health. Here's a book that answers the real question about Type 2 diabetes. This book is for recently diagnosed individuals with Type 2 diabetes or anyone ready to control their eating habits. Type 2 diabetics cookbook for beginners is a comprehensive, step-by-step introduction for people with type 2 diabetes. This book guides you through your diabetic journey, encouraging you to make healthy diet choices from the get-go. This book contains a 21-Day delicious and healthy meal plan that supports the quality of life for people with Type 2 diabetes through diet plans while improving the person's personal sense of control and well-being.

The simple recipes used in this book uphold the physiological health of people with type 2 diabetes by maintaining blood glucose as near normal as possible. Diabetes is preventable and can even be reversed. If you're already diagnosed with type 2 diabetes, it's never too late to make a positive change by eating healthier, exercising, and living a healthy lifestyle. Managing diabetes through diet doesn't mean living in deprivation; it means eating a delectable, balanced diet that will improve your mood and boost your energy. You don't resign yourself to a lifetime of tasteless food. This book contains some excellent diabetic diets, with plenty of delicious meals that wouldn't set your blood sugar soaring, helping you prepared to live a happy and well-nourished life despite being a diabetic.

What is Diabetes?

Diabetes is one of the leading causes of premature death in the United States. According to records, around 1.4 million new cases of diabetes are diagnosed each year, and an estimated 8 million people are undiagnosed or uninformed of their condition. The estimated number of people above 18 diagnosed and undiagnosed with diabetes is over 30.2 million. Diabetes is a disorder in which the body doesn't use the sugars in food in a typical way. The symptoms of diabetes in people differ, depending on the degree and complexity of the complication. When the body can't get sugar at the required place and time, it prompts elevated blood sugar levels in the circulatory system, leading to complications like nerve, kidney, eye, and cardiovascular disease.

Sugar (glucose) is the most preferred fuel for brain cells and muscle. However, it requires insulin to transport the glucose into cells for use. But when insulin levels are low, this means the insulin isn't sufficient to transport the sugar into the cells. This process prompts elevated blood sugar levels. Over the long run, the cells develop insulin resistance, and the attention now changes to the pancreas, which is required to make more insulin to move sugar into the cells; notwithstanding, more sugar is still left in the blood. Due to the pressure on the pancreas, it will eventually "wears out," which means it will no longer secrete enough insulin to move the sugar into the cells for energy.

Without continuous and careful management, diabetes can lead to life-threatening complications, including blindness and foot amputations, heart or kidney disease. It can lead to the development of sugars in the blood, increasing the risk of dangerous health complications, including stroke and heart disease.

What Causes Type 2 Diabetes?

The number of cases of Type 2 diabetes is soaring, related to the obesity epidemic. Type 2 diabetes occurs over time and involves problems getting enough sugar (glucose) into the body's cells. Overweight or obese is the greatest risk factor for Type 2 diabetes. However, the risk is higher if the concentration of weight is around the abdomen as opposed to the thighs and hips. The belly fat that surrounds the liver and abdominal organs are closely linked to insulin resistance. Calories obtained from everyday sugary drinks such as energy drinks, soda, coffee drinks, and processed foods like muffins, doughnuts, cereal, and candy could greatly increase the

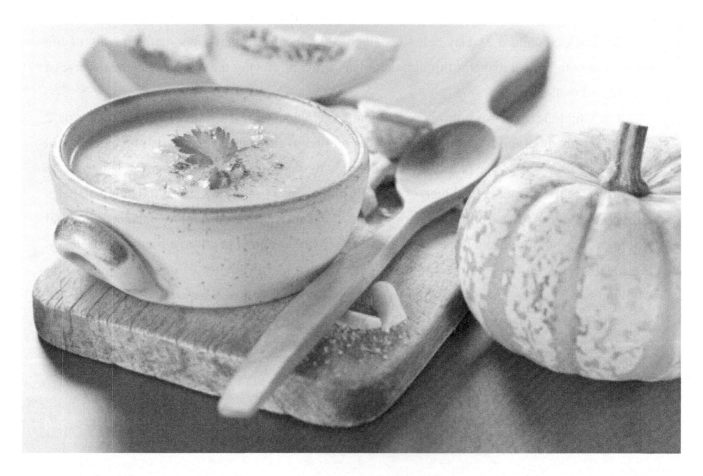

weight around your abdomen. In addition to eating healthy, cutting back on sugary foods can mean a slimmer waistline as well as a lower risk of diabetes.

Symptoms of Type 1&2 Diabetes include:

- Coma
- Itching
- Hunger
- Confusion
- Chest pain
- Headaches
- Blurry vision
- Extreme thirst
- Increased urination
- Fatigue or weakness
- Problems with gums
- Unexplained weight loss
- Problems having an erection
- Nausea, diarrhea, or constipation
- Numbness in the hands and feet

Diabetes is a troublesome disease to live with, regardless of how experienced you are. Adults diagnosed with Type 2 diabetes may have difficulties deciding what to eat and what not to eat. Indeed, even those who have lived with diabetes for quite some time could always use extra guidance and good dieting advice.

Differences Between Type 1 and Type 2 Diabetes

Most people know there are two types of diabetes, but not everyone understands the difference between them. The main difference between the two types of diabetes is that type 1 diabetes, also known as insulin-dependent diabetes, is an autoimmune disorder that often begins in childhood. It is a condition in which the immune system is attacking and destroying the insulin-producing cells in your pancreas, or the pancreas cells are not functioning effectively, leading to a reduction in the production of insulin. Without insulin, the glucose from carbohydrate foods cannot enter the cells. This causes glucose to build up in the blood, leaving your body's cells and tissues starved for energy.

Type 2, also known as adult-onset diabetes, is the most common form of diabetes. Type 2 diabetes is largely diet-related and can be caused by different factors. One factor that may cause this type of diabetes is when the pancreas begins to make less insulin. The second possible cause could be that the body becomes resistant to insulin. This means the pancreas is producing insulin, but the body doesn't use it efficiently. In both type 1 and type 2 diabetes, blood sugar levels can get too high because the body doesn't produce insulin or it does not utilize insulin properly. Diabetes can be managed, and diabetics patients can still live a relatively "normal" life.

How to Prevent Diabetes and Control Sugar Level.

Because type 1 diabetes is generic, blood tests are necessary for diagnosis. However, blood tests that determine the likelihood of type 1 can only be recommended by doctors when a patient begins to show symptoms. An A1C screening tests the blood sugar levels between two to three months and is typically used to diagnose type 1 and type 2 diabetes. Unlike type 1 diabetes which is generic, there are many ways to prevent type 2 diabetes. Ways to prevent type 2 diabetes include:

- Healthy diet
- Quit smoking

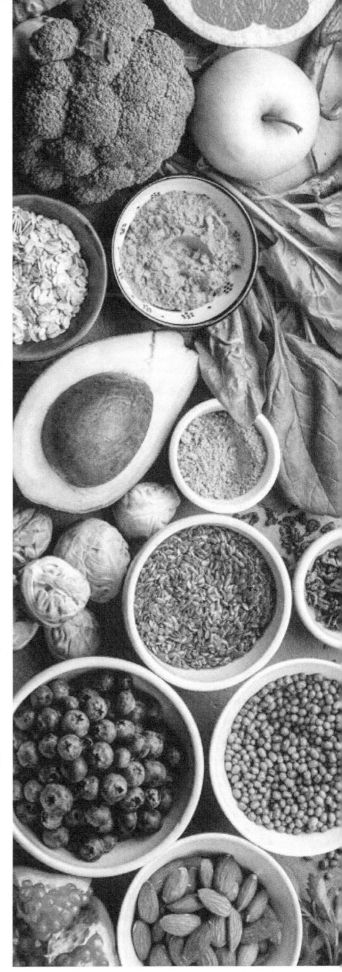

Introduction | 5

- Increase your fiber intake
- Exercise and weight management
- Maintain average blood pressure
- Maintain low alcohol consumption

Treatment for Diabetes

Type 1 diabetes has no cure; however, it can be managed by injecting insulin into the fatty tissue under the skin. The goal of Type 1 diabetic management is to maintain healthy blood glucose levels before and after meals. The patient needs to understand the required blood glucose requirement and maintain it at all times to experience good health and prevent or delay complications of diabetes. Different means of injecting insulin include:

- High-pressure air jet injector
- Syringe
- Insulin tub pump

Other measures needed to treat type 1 & 2 diabetes include

- Careful meal planning
- Healthy eating
- Healthy weight management
- Frequent blood sugar test
- Regular exercise
- Medications.
- Glucagon for emergency management of hypoglycemia

Additional Information Regarding Nutritional Goals for Type 2 Diabetic Patients

Carbohydrates

Dietary carbohydrates from vegetables, fruits, beans, starchy foods, cereals, bread, other grain products, legumes, vegetables, fruits, dairy products, and added sugars should provide the largest portion of an individual's energy requirements—both the amount consumed and the source of carbohydrate influence blood glucose and insulin responses. The terms "simple" and "complex" should not be used to classify carbohydrates because they do not help determine the impact of carbohydrates on blood glucose levels. Avoid fruit juices, canned fruits, or dried fruit and eat fresh fruits instead. You may eat fresh vegetables and frozen or canned vegetables.

Protein

Protein is found in poultry, meat, fish, beans, dairy products and some vegetables. Consume more of poultry and fish than red meat and trim extra fat from all meat. Avoid poultry skin. Choose nonfat or reduced-fat dairies, such as cheeses and yogurts. Current proof demonstrates individuals with diabetes have comparative protein prerequisites to those of everybody. Even though protein is important for the stimulation of insulin secretion, excess consumption may add to the pathogenesis of diabetic nephropathy.

Fats

Various studies indicate high-fat weight control diet can weaken glucose resistance and cause atherosclerotic heart disease, dyslipidemia, and obesity. Research likewise shows these equivalent metabolic anomalies are managed or improved by reducing saturated fat intake. Current suggestions on fat intake for everyone apply equally to individuals with diabetes. Reducing the intake of saturated fat by 10% or less and cholesterol intake to 300 mg/d or less. Research proposes monounsaturated fat (like nuts, fish, olive oil, canola oil, seeds, etc) may positively affect fatty oils and glycemic control in certain people with diabetes.

Sugars

In the past, sugar avoidance has been one of the major nutritional advice for people with diabetes. However, research has shown that sugars are an integral part of a healthy diet for diabetes, especially sugar gotten from vegetables, fruits, and dairy products. Added sugars, for example, sugar-sweetened and table sugar products, make up around 10% of the day-to-day energy needs. Refined sucrose gives a lower blood glucose reaction than many refined starches. Foods containing sugars vary in physiological effects and nutritional value. For example, sucrose and squeezed orange juice have comparative blood glucose effects but contain different nutrients and minerals. Consuming whole fruits and fruit juices causes blood glucose concentrations to peak slightly earlier but fall more quickly than consuming a comparable carbohydrate portion of white bread.

The Relationship Between Nutrients and Diabetes

People who have diabetes have excess sugar in their blood. Therefore, managing diabetes means managing your blood sugar level through the consumption of food rich in certain nutrients or through insulin injection. The nutrients in what you eat is connected your overall well-being. The right nutrient choices will help you control your blood sugar level. Eating food reach in the right nutrients is one of the primary things you can do to help control diabetes. There isn't one specific "diabetes diet" for people suffering from diabetes. but a dietician can work with you to design a meal plan to guide you on what kinds of food to eat and what snacks to have at mealtimes. A nutritious diet consists of:

- 20% calories from protein
- 30% or lesser calories from fat
- 40% - 60% from carbohydrates.

Your diet should also be low in salt, cholesterol, and added sugar.

Contrary to belief eating some sugar doesn't cause problems for most people who have diabetes. However, it's important to watch the amount of sugar you consume and make sure it's part of a balanced diet.

In general, each meal should have the following nutrients:

- 2 - 5 choices (or up to 60 grams) of carbohydrates
- A certain amount of fat
- One choice of protein

What to Eat:

- Healthy nuts fats such as almonds, olive oil, walnuts, cashews and peanuts.
- Fish and shellfish.
- Organic chicken or turkey.
- Fresh fruits, vegetables, and whole fruit.
- Protein from eggs, low-fat dairy, beans, and unsweetened yogurt.
- High-fiber cereals and slices of bread made from whole grains.

What to Avoid:

- Processed or fast food, especially those high in sugar.
- Red or processed meat.
- Sugary cereals, white bread, refined pasta, or rice.
- Low-fat products with added sugar, such as fat-free yogurt.

Besides providing diets that will help you manage type 2 diabetes, just like Delicious Dish for Diabetics: Eating Well with Type 2 Diabetes by Robin Ellis, this book offers other benefits as well. The real meat in this book is its use of simple sentences to explain diabetes-related topics such as understand type 2 diabetes, design a menu, how much food should be eaten in a day, food to eat and avoid, and a healthy meal plan for Type 2 diabetes patient. If you are recently diagnosed with Type 2 diabetes, you need a book like this to help get you on the right track for healthy living.

Carbohydrate counting is going to be part of your life now. The recipes in this book are made up of generous amounts of fruits, vegetables, and fiber, which are likely to reduce the risk of cardiovascular diseases and certain types of cancer. The recipes in these book are similar to what you will find in The American Diabetes Association Diabetes Comfort Food Cookbook by Robin Webb, M.S. Embracing a healthy eating plan is the best and fastest way to keep your blood glucose level under control and prevent diabetes complications. Type 2 Diabetics Cookbook for Beginners is here to help you navigate your way around diabetes management by providing a 21-day meal plan made from 200 delicious and healthy recipes to help you develop a good eating habit and ultimately manage your diabetes.

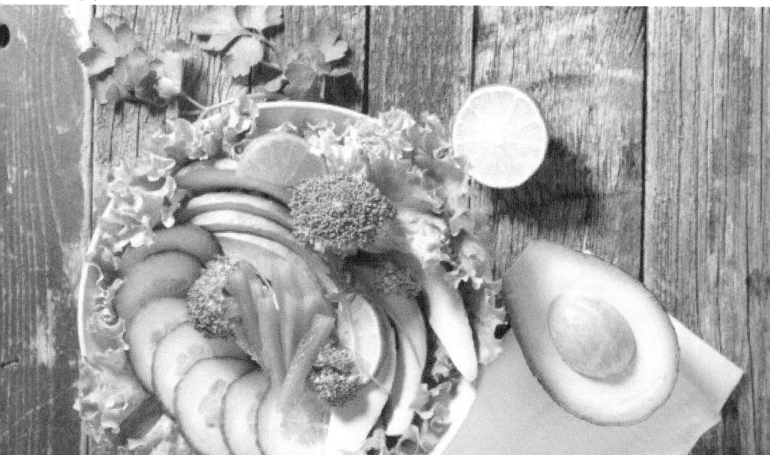

Chapter 1 Breakfasts

Lentil, Squash, and Tomato Omelet   9

Blueberry Cornmeal Muffins   9

Spinach and Feta Egg Bake   9

Cinnamon Overnight Oats   9

Two-Cheese Grits   9

Blueberry-Chia Smoothie   10

Baked Avocado and Egg   10

Berry–French Toast Stratas   10

Asparagus and Bell Pepper Strata   10

Golden Potato Cakes   10

Toads In Holes   11

Coddled Huevos Rancheros   11

Veggie And Egg White Scramble With Pepper

Jack Cheese   11

Ratatouille Baked Eggs   11

Pumpkin Spice Muffins   12

Spicy Tomato Smoothie   12

Tofu, Kale, and Mushroom Breakfast

Scramble   12

Whole-Grain Strawberry Pancakes   12

Grain-Free Applesauce Crêpes   12

Easy Breakfast Chia Pudding   13

Blueberry Coconut Breakfast Cookies   13

Ginger Blackberry Bliss Smoothie Bowl   13

Creamy Blueberry Quesadillas   13

Sweet Potato Toasts   13

Creamy Green Smoothie   13

Gouda Egg Casserole   14

Shredded Potato Omelet   14

Pumpkin–Peanut Butter Single-Serve

Muffins   14

Easy Sweet Potato and Egg Sandwiches   14

Hoe Cakes   15

Breakfast Hash   15

Cinnamon French Toast   15

Hash Browns   15

Breakfast Casserole   15

Mandarin Orange–Millet Breakfast Bowl   16

Bran Apple Muffins   16

Sweet Potato Breakfast Bites   16

Savory Grits   16

Pumpkin Apple Waffles   17

Black Bean Breakfast Burrito   17

Easy Buckwheat Crêpes   17

Goji Berry Muesli   17

Breakfast Meatballs   17

Cauliflower Scramble   18

Crepe Cakes   18

Low-Carb Peanut Butter Pancakes   18

Egg Bites with Sausage and Peppers   18

Lentil, Squash, and Tomato Omelet

Prep time: 5 minutes | Cook time: 45 minutes | Serves 2

1 cup water
⅓ cup dried lentils, picked over, rinsed, and drained
Extra-virgin olive oil cooking spray
1 medium zucchini, thinly sliced
½ cup grape tomatoes, coarsely chopped
1 garlic clove, chopped
2 tablespoons chopped fresh chives
2 large eggs
2 tablespoons nonfat milk

1. Preheat the oven to 350°F. 2. In a small saucepan set over high heat, heat the water until it boils. 3. Add the lentils. Reduce the heat to low. Simmer for about 15 minutes, or until most of the liquid has been absorbed. In a colander, drain and set aside. 4. Lightly coat an 8- or 9-inch nonstick skillet with cooking spray. Place the skillet over medium-high heat. 5. Add the zucchini, tomatoes, garlic, and chives. Sauté for 5 to 10 minutes, stirring frequently, or until soft. 6. Add the lentils to the skillet. 7. In a medium bowl, beat together the eggs and milk with a fork. 8. Lightly coat a small casserole or baking dish with cooking spray. 9. In the bottom of the prepared dish, spread the vegetable mixture. 10. Pour the egg mixture over. Use a fork to distribute evenly. 11. Place the dish in the preheated oven. Bake for 15 to 20 minutes, or until the dish is set in the middle. 12. Slice in half and enjoy!

Per Serving

Calories: 209 | fat: 6g | protein: 16g | carbs: 25g | sugars: 4g | fiber: 5g | sodium: 90mg

Blueberry Cornmeal Muffins

Prep time: 5 minutes | Cook time: 25 minutes | Makes 12 muffins

2 cups oat flour
½ cup fine corn flour
¼ cup coconut sugar
2 teaspoons baking powder
½ teaspoon baking soda
¼ teaspoon sea salt
1 teaspoon lemon zest
½ cup + 2–3 tablespoons plain nondairy yogurt
¼ cup pure maple syrup
½ cup plain low-fat nondairy milk
1 teaspoon lemon juice or apple cider vinegar
1 cup frozen or fresh blueberries
1 tablespoon oat flour

1. Preheat the oven to 350°F. Line a muffin pan with 12 parchment cupcake liners. 2. In a large bowl, combine the oat flour, corn flour, sugar, baking powder, baking soda, salt, and lemon zest. Stir well. In a medium bowl, combine the yogurt, syrup, milk, and lemon juice or apple cider vinegar, and stir to combine. Add the wet ingredients to the dry and mix until just combined. Toss the berries with the oat flour, and fold them into the batter. Spoon the batter into the muffin liners. Bake for 25 minutes. Remove from the oven and let the muffins cool in the pan for a couple of minutes, then transfer to a cooling rack.

Per Serving 1 muffin:

calorie: 152 | fat: 2g | protein: 4g | carbs: 31g | sugars: 11g | fiber: 3g | sodium: 191mg

Spinach and Feta Egg Bake

Prep time: 7 minutes | Cook time: 23 to 25 minutes | Serves 2

Avocado oil spray
⅓ cup diced red onion
1 cup frozen chopped spinach, thawed and drained
4 large eggs
¼ cup heavy (whipping) cream
Sea salt and freshly ground black pepper, to taste
¼ teaspoon cayenne pepper
½ cup crumbled feta cheese
¼ cup shredded Parmesan cheese

1. Spray a deep pan with oil. Put the onion in the pan, and place the pan in the air fryer basket. Set the air fryer to 350°F (177°C) and bake for 7 minutes. 2. Sprinkle the spinach over the onion. 3. In a medium bowl, beat the eggs, heavy cream, salt, black pepper, and cayenne. Pour this mixture over the vegetables. 4. Top with the feta and Parmesan cheese. Bake for 16 to 18 minutes, until the eggs are set and lightly brown.

Per Serving

Calories: 366 | fat: 26g | protein: 25g | carbs: 8g | sugars: 4g | fiber: 3g | sodium: 520mg

Cinnamon Overnight Oats

Prep time: 5 Minutes | Cook Time: 0 Minutes | Serves 1

⅓ cup unsweetened almond milk
⅓ cup rolled oats (use gluten-free if necessary)
¼ apple, cored and finely
chopped
2 tablespoons chopped walnuts
½ teaspoon cinnamon
Pinch sea salt

1. In a single-serving container or mason jar, combine all of the ingredients and mix well. 2. Cover and refrigerate overnight.

Per Serving

Calories: 358 | fat: 14g | protein: 13g | carbs: 47g | sugars: 10g | fiber: 9g | sodium: 213mg

Two-Cheese Grits

Prep time: 10 minutes | Cook time: 10 to 12 minutes | Serves 4

⅔ cup instant grits
1 teaspoon salt
1 teaspoon freshly ground black pepper
¾ cup milk, whole or 2%
1 large egg, beaten
3 ounces (85 g) cream cheese, at room temperature
1 tablespoon butter, melted
1 cup shredded mild Cheddar cheese
1 to 2 tablespoons oil

1. In a large bowl, combine the grits, salt, and pepper. Stir in the milk, egg, cream cheese, and butter until blended. Stir in the Cheddar cheese. 2. Preheat the air fryer to 400°F (204°C). Spritz a baking pan with oil. 3. Pour the grits mixture into the prepared pan and place it in the air fryer basket. 4. Cook for 5 minutes. Stir the mixture and cook for 5 minutes more for soupy grits or 7 minutes more for firmer grits.

Per Serving

Calories: 302 | fat: 18g | protein: 13g | carbs: 21g | sugars: 4g | fiber: 1g | sodium: 621mg

Blueberry-Chia Smoothie

Prep time: 5 minutes | Cook time: 0 minutes | Serves 2

2 cups frozen blueberries
½ medium frozen banana
2 tablespoons peanut butter

2 tablespoons chia seeds
12 ounces unsweetened soy milk, plus extra if needed

1. Combine the blueberries, banana, peanut butter, chia seeds, and soy milk in a blender and blend on high speed until smooth. Use a spatula to scrape down the sides as needed. 2. Serve immediately. If it's too thick, add more soy milk or water by the tablespoonful until you've reached the desired consistency.

Per Serving

Calories: 249 | fat: 10g | protein: 10g | carbs: 35g | sugars: 17g | fiber: 8g | sodium: 181mg

Baked Avocado and Egg

Prep time: 10 minutes | Cook time: 10 minutes | Serves 2

1 large avocado, halved and pitted
2 large eggs
2 tomato slices, divided

½ cup nonfat cottage cheese, divided
Fresh cilantro, for garnish

1. Preheat the oven to 425°F. 2. Slice a thin piece from the bottom of each avocado half so they sit flat. 3. Remove a small amount from each avocado half to make a bigger hole to hold the egg. 4. On a small foil-lined baking sheet, place the halves hollow-side up. 5. Break 1 egg into each half. 6. Top each with 1 slice of tomato and ¼ cup of cottage cheese. 7. Place the sheet in the preheated oven. Bake for 8 to 10 minutes for softboiled consistency, or longer for a firmer egg. 8. Garnish with fresh cilantro and serve.

Per Serving

Calories: 262 | fat: 20g | protein: 12g | carbs: 12g | sugars: 2g | fiber: 7g | sodium: 214mg

Berry-French Toast Stratas

Prep time: 15 minutes | Cook time: 20 to 25 minutes | Serves 6

3 cups assorted fresh berries, such as blueberries, raspberries or cut-up strawberries
1 tablespoon granulated sugar
4 cups cubes (¾ inch) whole wheat bread (about 5 slices)
1½ cups fat-free egg product or 6 eggs

½ cup fat-free (skim) milk
½ cup fat-free half-and-half
2 tablespoons honey
1½ teaspoons vanilla
1 teaspoon ground cinnamon
¼ teaspoon ground nutmeg
½ teaspoon powdered sugar, if desired

1. In medium bowl, mix fruit and granulated sugar; set aside. 2. Heat oven to 350°F. Spray 12 regular-size muffin cups generously with cooking spray. Divide bread cubes evenly among muffin cups. 3. In large bowl, beat remaining ingredients, except powdered sugar, with fork or whisk until well mixed. Pour egg mixture over bread cubes, pushing down lightly with spoon to soak bread cubes. (If all egg mixture doesn't fit into cups, let cups stand up to 10 minutes, gradually adding remaining egg mixture as bread cubes soak it up.) 4. Bake 20 to 25 minutes or until centers are set. Cool 5 minutes. Remove from muffin cups, placing 2 stratas on each of 6 plates. Divide fruit mixture evenly over stratas; sprinkle with powdered sugar.

Per Serving

Calories: 218 | fat: 6g | protein: 11g | carbs: 32g | sugars: 17g | fiber: 4g | sodium: 216mg

Asparagus and Bell Pepper Strata

Prep time: 10 minutes | Cook time: 14 to 20 minutes | Serves 4

8 large asparagus spears, trimmed and cut into 2-inch pieces
⅓ cup shredded carrot
½ cup chopped red bell pepper
2 slices low-sodium whole-

wheat bread, cut into ½-inch cubes
3 egg whites
1 egg
3 tablespoons 1% milk
½ teaspoon dried thyme

1. In a baking pan, combine the asparagus, carrot, red bell pepper, and 1 tablespoon of water. Bake in the air fryer at 330°F (166°C) for 3 to 5 minutes, or until crisp-tender. Drain well. 2. Add the bread cubes to the vegetables and gently toss. 3. In a medium bowl, whisk the egg whites, egg, milk, and thyme until frothy. 4. Pour the egg mixture into the pan. Bake for 11 to 15 minutes, or until the strata is slightly puffy and set and the top starts to brown. Serve.

Per Serving

Calories: 92 | fat: 2g | protein: 8g | carbs: 11g | sugars: 3g | fiber: 3g | sodium: 142mg

Golden Potato Cakes

Prep time: 10 minutes | Cook time: 25 minutes | Serves 4

½ pound russet potatoes, peeled, shredded, rinsed, and patted dry
¼ sweet onion, chopped
1 teaspoon extra-virgin olive oil

1 teaspoon chopped fresh thyme
Sea salt
Freshly ground black pepper
Nonstick cooking spray
1 cup unsweetened applesauce

1. Place the potatoes, onion, oil, and thyme in a large bowl and stir to mix well. 2. Season the potato mixture generously with salt and pepper. 3. Place a large skillet over medium heat and lightly coat it with cooking spray. 4. Scoop about ¼ cup of potato mixture per cake into the skillet and press down with a spatula, about 4 cakes per batch. 5. Cook until the bottoms are golden brown and firm, about 5 to 7 minutes, then flip the cake over. Cook the other side until it is golden brown and the cake is completely cooked through, about 5 minutes more. 6. Remove the cakes to a plate and repeat with the remaining mixture. 7. Serve with the applesauce.

Per Serving

Calories: 88 | fat: 1g | protein: 1g | carbs: 19g | sugars: 7g | fiber: 2g | sodium: 6mg

Toads In Holes

Prep time: 5 minutes | Cook time: 5 minutes | Serves 2

2 tablespoons butter
2 slices whole-wheat bread
2 large eggs

Sea salt
Freshly ground black pepper

1. In a medium nonstick skillet over medium heat, heat the butter until it bubbles. 2. As the butter heats, cut a 3-inch hole in the middle of each piece of bread. Discard the centers. 3. Place the bread pieces in the butter in the pan. Carefully crack an egg into the hole of each piece of bread. 4. Cook until the bread crisps and the egg whites set, about 3 minutes. 5. Flip and cook just until the yolk is almost set, 1 to 2 minutes more. 6. Season to taste with the salt and pepper.

Per Serving

Calories: 254 | fat: 17g | protein: 10g | carbs: 14g | sugars: 2g | fiber: 2g | sodium: 218mg

Coddled Huevos Rancheros

Prep time: 5 minutes | Cook time: 10 minutes | Serves 2

2 teaspoons unsalted butter
4 large eggs
1 cup drained cooked black beans, or two-thirds 15-ounce can black beans, rinsed and drained
Two 7-inch corn or whole-wheat tortillas, warmed

½ cup chunky tomato salsa (such as Pace brand)
2 cups shredded romaine lettuce
1 tablespoon chopped fresh cilantro
2 tablespoons grated Cotija cheese

1. Pour 1 cup water into the Instant Pot and place a long-handled silicone steam rack into the pot. (If you don't have the long-handled rack, use the wire metal steam rack and a homemade sling) 2. Coat each of four 4-ounce ramekins with ½ teaspoon butter. Crack an egg into each ramekin. Place the ramekins on the steam rack in the pot. 3. Secure the lid and set the Pressure Release to Sealing. Select the Steam setting and set the cooking time for 3 minutes at low pressure. (The pot will take about 5 minutes to come up to pressure before the cooking program begins.) 4. While the eggs are cooking, in a small saucepan over low heat, warm the beans for about 5 minutes, stirring occasionally. Cover the saucepan and remove from the heat. (Alternatively, warm the beans in a covered bowl in a microwave for 1 minute. Leave the beans covered until ready to serve.) 5. When the cooking program ends, let the pressure release naturally for 5 minutes, then move the Pressure Release to Venting to release any remaining steam. Open the pot and, wearing heat-resistant mitts, grasp the handles of the steam rack and carefully lift it out of the pot. 6. Place a warmed tortilla on each plate and spoon ½ cup of the beans onto each tortilla. Run a knife around the inside edge of each ramekin to loosen the egg and unmold two eggs onto the beans on each tortilla. Spoon the salsa over the eggs and top with the lettuce, cilantro, and cheese. Serve right away.

Per Serving

Calorie: 112 | fat: 8g | protein: 8g | carbs: 3g | sugars: 0g | fiber: 0g | sodium: 297mg

Veggie And Egg White Scramble With Pepper Jack Cheese

Prep time: 5 minutes | Cook time: 10 minutes | Serves 2

2 tablespoons extra-virgin olive oil
½ red onion, finely chopped
1 green bell pepper, seeded and finely chopped
8 large egg whites (or 4 whole

large eggs), beaten
½ teaspoon sea salt
2 ounces grated pepper Jack cheese
Salsa (optional, for serving)

1. In a medium nonstick skillet over medium-high heat, heat the olive oil until it shimmers. 2. Add the onion and bell pepper and cook, stirring occasionally, until the vegetables begin to brown, about 5 minutes. 3. Meanwhile, in a small bowl, whisk together the egg whites and salt. 4. Add the egg whites to the pan and cook, stirring, until the whites set, about 3 minutes. Add the cheese. Cook, stirring, 1 minute more. 5. Serve topped with salsa, if desired.

Per Serving

Calories: 320 | fat: 23g | protein: 22g | carbs: 7g | sugars: 4g | fiber: 2g | sodium: 584mg

Ratatouille Baked Eggs

Prep time: 20 minutes | Cook time: 50 minutes | Serves 4

2 teaspoons extra-virgin olive oil
½ sweet onion, finely chopped
2 teaspoons minced garlic
½ small eggplant, peeled and diced
1 green zucchini, diced
1 yellow zucchini, diced
1 red bell pepper, seeded and diced

3 tomatoes, seeded and chopped
1 tablespoon chopped fresh oregano
1 tablespoon chopped fresh basil
Pinch red pepper flakes
Sea salt
Freshly ground black pepper
4 large eggs

1. Preheat the oven to 350°F. 2. Place a large ovenproof skillet over medium heat and add the olive oil. 3. Sauté the onion and garlic until softened and translucent, about 3 minutes. Stir in the eggplant and sauté for about 10 minutes, stirring occasionally. Stir in the zucchini and pepper and sauté for 5 minutes. 4. Reduce the heat to low and cover. Cook until the vegetables are soft, about 15 minutes. 5. Stir in the tomatoes, oregano, basil, and red pepper flakes, and cook 10 minutes more. Season the ratatouille with salt and pepper. 6. Use a spoon to create four wells in the mixture. Crack an egg into each well. 7. Place the skillet in the oven and bake until the eggs are firm, about 5 minutes. 8. Remove from the oven. Serve the eggs with a generous scoop of vegetables.

Per Serving

Calories: 164 | fat: 8g | protein: 10g | carbs: 16g | sugars: 8g | fiber: 5g | sodium: 275mg

Pumpkin Spice Muffins

Prep time: 10 minutes | Cook time: 15 minutes | Serves 6

1 cup blanched finely ground almond flour
½ cup granular erythritol
½ teaspoon baking powder
¼ cup unsalted butter, softened
¼ cup pure pumpkin purée
½ teaspoon ground cinnamon
¼ teaspoon ground nutmeg
1 teaspoon vanilla extract
2 large eggs

1. In a large bowl, mix almond flour, erythritol, baking powder, butter, pumpkin purée, cinnamon, nutmeg, and vanilla. 2. Gently stir in eggs. 3. Evenly pour the batter into six silicone muffin cups. Place muffin cups into the air fryer basket, working in batches if necessary. 4. Adjust the temperature to 300ºF (149ºC) and bake for 15 minutes. 5. When completely cooked, a toothpick inserted in center will come out mostly clean. Serve warm.

Per Serving

Calories: 261 | fat: 19g | protein: 8g | carbs: 16g | sugars: 11g | fiber: 3g | sodium: 34mg

Spicy Tomato Smoothie

Prep time: 5 minutes | Cook time: 0 minutes | Serves 2

1 cup tomato juice
2 tomatoes, diced
¼ English cucumber
Juice of 1 lemon
1 teaspoon hot sauce
4 ice cubes

1. Put the tomato juice, tomatoes, cucumber, lemon juice, hot sauce, and ice cubes in a blender and blend until smooth. 2. Pour into two glasses and serve.

Per Serving

Calories: 51 | fat: 1g | protein: 2g | carbs: 11g | sugars: 7g | fiber: 2g | sodium: 34mg

Tofu, Kale, and Mushroom Breakfast Scramble

Prep time: 5 minutes | Cook time: 10 minutes | Serves 2

2 tablespoons extra-virgin olive oil
½ red onion, finely chopped
8 ounces mushrooms, sliced
1 cup chopped kale
8 ounces tofu, cut into pieces
2 garlic cloves, minced
Pinch red pepper flakes
½ teaspoon sea salt
⅛ teaspoon freshly ground black pepper

1. In a medium nonstick skillet over medium-high heat, heat the olive oil until it shimmers. 2. Add the onion, mushrooms, and kale. Cook, stirring occasionally, until the vegetables begin to brown, about 5 minutes. 3. Add the tofu. Cook, stirring, until the tofu starts to brown, 3 to 4 minutes more. 4. Add the garlic, red pepper flakes, salt, and pepper. Cook, stirring constantly, for 30 seconds more.

Per Serving

Calories: 234 | fat: 18g | protein: 12g | carbs: 10g | sugars: 4g | fiber: 2g | sodium: 601mg

Whole-Grain Strawberry Pancakes

Prep time: 30 minutes | Cook time: 10 minutes | Serves 7

1½ cups whole wheat flour
3 tablespoons sugar
1 teaspoon baking powder
½ teaspoon baking soda
½ teaspoon salt
3 eggs or ¾ cup fat-free egg product
1 container (6 ounces) vanilla
low-fat yogurt
¾ cup water
3 tablespoons canola oil
1¾ cups sliced fresh strawberries
1 container (6 ounces) strawberry low-fat yogurt

1. Heat griddle to 375°F or heat 12-inch skillet over medium heat. Grease with canola oil if necessary (or spray with cooking spray before heating). 2. In large bowl, mix flour, sugar, baking powder, baking soda and salt; set aside. In medium bowl, beat eggs, vanilla yogurt, water and oil with egg beater or whisk until well blended. Pour egg mixture all at once into flour mixture; stir until moistened. 3. For each pancake, pour slightly less than ¼ cup batter onto hot griddle. Cook pancakes 1 to 2 minutes or until bubbly on top, puffed and dry around edges. Turn; cook other sides 1 to 2 minutes or until golden brown. 4. Top each serving with ¼ cup sliced strawberries and 1 to 2 tablespoons strawberry yogurt.

Per Serving

Calories: 260 | fat: 9g | protein: 8g | carbs: 34g | sugars: 13g | fiber: 4g | sodium: 380mg

Grain-Free Applesauce Crêpes

Prep time: 5 minutes | Cook time: 10 minutes | Serves 2

½ cup liquid egg substitute
½ cup coconut flour
¾ cup unsweetened vanilla almond milk
1 teaspoon vanilla extract
1 teaspoon granulated stevia
Pinch salt
Extra-virgin olive oil cooking spray
½ cup unsweetened applesauce
½ cup nonfat cottage cheese
Ground cinnamon

1. To a blender, add the egg substitute, coconut flour, vanilla almond milk, vanilla, stevia, and salt. Process until thoroughly mixed. 2. Place a nonstick skillet set over medium-high heat. Coat with cooking spray. 3. When the pan is hot, pour in a one-half of the batter. Swirl to evenly coat the bottom of the pan. Cook for about 2 minutes, or until the top is set and the bottom is light brown. 4. Using a silicone spatula, loosen the top edge of the crêpe. Tilting the pan, roll the crêpe toward the bottom of the pan. Remove from the pan and set aside. Repeat with the remaining batter. 5. In a small, covered microwave-safe bowl, gently warm the applesauce in the microwave on medium for about 30 seconds. 6. Remove from the microwave. Add the cottage cheese. Mix gently until blended. 7. Divide the crêpes between 2 plates. 8. Top each with ½ cup of the applesauce–cottage cheese mixture. 9. Sprinkle with cinnamon and serve immediately.

Per Serving

Calories: 169 | fat: 6g | protein: 11g | carbs: 19g | sugars: 13g | fiber: 3g | sodium: 315mg

Easy Breakfast Chia Pudding

Prep time: 5 minutes | Cook time: 0 minutes | Serves 4

4 cups unsweetened almond milk or skim milk
¾ cup chia seeds
1 teaspoon ground cinnamon
Pinch sea salt

1. Stir together the milk, chia seeds, cinnamon, and salt in a medium bowl. 2. Cover the bowl with plastic wrap and chill in the refrigerator until the pudding is thick, about 1 hour. 3. Sweeten with your favorite sweetener and fruit.

Per Serving

Calories: 129 | fat: 3g | protein: 10g | carbs: 16g | sugars: 12g | fiber: 3g | sodium: 131mg

Blueberry Coconut Breakfast Cookies

Prep time: 10 minutes | Cook time: 15 minutes | Serves 4

4 tablespoons unsalted butter, at room temperature
2 medium bananas
4 large eggs
½ cup unsweetened applesauce
1 teaspoon vanilla extract
⅔ cup coconut flour
¼ teaspoon salt
1 cup fresh or frozen blueberries

1. Preheat the oven to 375ºF. 2. In a medium bowl, mash the butter and bananas together with a fork until combined. The bananas can be a little chunky. 3. Add the eggs, applesauce, and vanilla to the bananas and mix well. 4. Stir in the coconut flour and salt. 5. Gently fold in the blueberries. 6. Drop about 2 tablespoons of dough on a baking sheet for each cookie and flatten it a bit with the back of a spoon. Bake for about 13 minutes, or until firm to the touch.

Per Serving

Calories: 263 | fat: 15g | protein: 8g | carbs: 24g | sugars: 14g | fiber: 4g | sodium: 225mg

Ginger Blackberry Bliss Smoothie Bowl

Prep time: 5 minutes | Cook time: 0 minutes | Serves 2

½ cup frozen blackberries
1 cup plain Greek yogurt
1 cup baby spinach
½ cup unsweetened almond
milk
½ teaspoon peeled and grated fresh ginger
¼ cup chopped pecans

1. In a blender or food processor, combine the blackberries, yogurt, spinach, almond milk, and ginger. Blend until smooth. 2. Spoon the mixture into two bowls. 3. Top each bowl with 2 tablespoons of chopped pecans and serve.

Per Serving

Calories: 211 | fat: 11g | protein: 10g | carbs: 18g | sugars: 13g | fiber: 4g | sodium: 149mg

Creamy Blueberry Quesadillas

Prep time: 5 minutes | Cook time: 5 minutes | Serves 2

¼ cup plain nonfat Greek yogurt
¼ cup nonfat ricotta cheese
2 tablespoons finely ground flaxseed
½ teaspoon cinnamon
¼ teaspoon vanilla extract
1 tablespoon granulated stevia
2 (8-inch) low-carb whole-wheat tortillas
½ cup fresh blueberries, divided

1. Preheat the oven to 400°F. 2. Line a baking dish with aluminum foil. 3. In a small bowl, mix together the yogurt, ricotta cheese, flaxseed, cinnamon, vanilla, and stevia. 4. Place the tortillas in the baking dish. 5. Spread half of the yogurt mixture on each tortilla, almost to the edges. 6. Top each with ¼ cup of blueberries. Fold the tortillas in half. 7. Place the dish in the preheated oven. Bake for 3 to 4 minutes. 8. Enjoy immediately!

Per Serving

Calories: 221 | fat: 7g | protein: 9g | carbs: 31g | sugars: 8g | fiber: 7g | sodium: 308mg

Sweet Potato Toasts

Prep time: 10 minutes | Cook time: 2 minutes | Serves 1

2 slices sprouted grain bread
½ cup mashed cooked sweet potato, peel removed
½–1 teaspoon lemon juice
A couple pinches of sea salt
Freshly ground black pepper (optional)
2 tablespoons cubed avocado or 1 tablespoon sliced black olives

1. Toast the bread. In a small bowl, mash the sweet potato with the lemon juice (adjusting to taste), salt, and pepper (if using). Distribute the mashed sweet potato between the slices of toast, and top with either the cubed avocado or the black olives. Serve!

Per Serving

Calorie: 312 | fat: 5g | protein: 8g | carbs: 40g | sugars: 11g | fiber: 8g | sodium: 1018mg

Creamy Green Smoothie

Prep time: 5 minutes | Cook time: 0 minutes | Serves 2

2 cups shredded kale
½ avocado, diced
½ Granny Smith apple, unpeeled, cored and chopped
1 cup unsweetened almond
milk
¼ cup 2 percent plain Greek yogurt
3 ice cubes

1. Put the kale, avocado, apple, almond milk, yogurt, and ice in a blender and blend until smooth and thick. 2. Pour into two glasses and serve.

Per Serving

Calories: 153 | fat: 9g | protein: 4g | carbs: 15g | sugars: 7g | fiber: 6g | sodium: 117mg

Gouda Egg Casserole

Prep time: 12 minutes | Cook time: 20 minutes | Serves 4

Nonstick cooking spray
1 slice whole grain bread, toasted
½ cup shredded smoked Gouda cheese
6 large eggs
¼ cup half-and-half
¼ teaspoon kosher salt
¼ teaspoon freshly ground black pepper
¼ teaspoon dry mustard

1. Spray a 6-inch cake pan with cooking spray, or if the pan is nonstick, skip this step. If you don't have a 6-inch cake pan, any bowl or pan that fits inside your pressure cooker should work. 2. Crumble the toast into the bottom of the pan. Sprinkle with the cheese. 3. In a medium bowl, whisk together the eggs, half-and-half, salt, pepper, and dry mustard. 4. Pour the egg mixture into the pan. Loosely cover the pan with aluminum foil. 5. Pour 1½ cups water into the electric pressure cooker and insert a wire rack or trivet. Place the covered pan on top of the rack. 6. Close and lock the lid of the pressure cooker. Set the valve to sealing. 7. Cook on high pressure for 20 minutes. 8. When the cooking is complete, hit Cancel and quick release the pressure. 9. Once the pin drops, unlock and remove the lid. 10. Carefully transfer the pan from the pressure cooker to a cooling rack and let it sit for 5 minutes. 11. Cut into 4 wedges and serve.

Per Serving

Calories: 217 | fat: 13g | protein: 18g | carbs: 7g | sugars: 1g | fiber: 1g | sodium: 562mg

Shredded Potato Omelet

Prep time: 15 minutes | Cook time: 20 minutes | Serves 6

2 cups shredded cooked potatoes
¼ cup minced onion
¼ cup minced green bell pepper
1 cup egg substitute
¼ cup fat-free milk
¼ teaspoon salt
⅛ teaspoon black pepper
1 cup 75%-less-fat shredded cheddar cheese
1 cup water

1. With nonstick cooking spray, spray the inside of a round baking dish that will fit in your Instant Pot inner pot. 2. Sprinkle the potatoes, onion, and bell pepper around the bottom of the baking dish. 3. Mix together the egg substitute, milk, salt, and pepper in mixing bowl. Pour over potato mixture. 4. Top with cheese. 5. Add water, place the steaming rack into the bottom of the inner pot and then place the round baking dish on top. 6. Close the lid and secure to the locking position. Be sure the vent is turned to sealing. Set for 20 minutes on Manual at high pressure. 7. Let the pressure release naturally. 8. Carefully remove the baking dish with the handles of the steaming rack and allow to stand 10 minutes before cutting and serving.

Per Serving

Calories: 130 | fat: 3g | protein: 12g | carbs: 13g | sugars: 2g | fiber: 2g | sodium: 415mg

Pumpkin–Peanut Butter Single-Serve Muffins

Prep time: 10 minutes | Cook time: 25 minutes | Serves 2

2 tablespoons powdered peanut butter
2 tablespoons coconut flour
2 tablespoons finely ground flaxseed
1 teaspoon pumpkin pie spice
½ teaspoon baking powder
1 tablespoon dried cranberries
½ cup water
1 cup canned pumpkin
2 large eggs
½ teaspoon vanilla extract
Extra-virgin olive oil cooking spray

1. Preheat the oven to 350°F. 2. In a medium bowl, stir together the powdered peanut butter, coconut flour, flaxseed, pumpkin pie spice, baking powder, dried cranberries, and water. 3. In a separate medium bowl, whisk together the pumpkin and eggs until smooth. 4. Add the pumpkin mixture to the dry ingredients. Stir to combine. 5. Add the vanilla. Mix together well. 6. Spray 2 (8-ounce) ramekins with cooking spray. 7. Spoon half of the batter into each ramekin. 8. Place the ramekins on a baking and carefully transfer the sheet to the preheated oven. Bake for 25 minutes, or until a toothpick in the center comes out clean. Enjoy immediately!

Per Serving

Calories: 286 | fat: 16g | protein: 15g | carbs: 24g | sugars: 9g | fiber: 7g | sodium: 189mg

Easy Sweet Potato and Egg Sandwiches

Prep time: 5 minutes | Cook time: 10 minutes | Serves 2

1 large sweet potato, sliced into 4 (¼-inch [6-mm]-thick) rounds
2 ounces (57 g) shredded
mozzarella cheese
Cooking oil spray, as needed
2 large eggs

1. Preheat the oven to broil. Line a large baking sheet with parchment paper. 2. Arrange the sweet potato rounds evenly on the prepared baking sheet. Broil the sweet potatoes for 4 to 6 minutes, until they are beginning to brown. Make sure to keep an eye on them so they don't burn. 3. Remove the sweet potatoes from the oven and add 1 ounce (28 g) of mozzarella cheese per sweet potato round to two of the rounds. Remove the plain sweet potato rounds from the baking sheet, and return the baking sheet with the cheese-topped sweet potatoes to the oven. Broil the rounds for 1 to 2 minutes, until the cheese begins to brown. 4. Remove the baking sheet from the oven and set it aside with the other sweet potato rounds. 5. Heat a medium skillet over medium heat. Spray it with the cooking oil spray and add the eggs. Scramble the eggs to your preferred doneness. 6. Top the cheesy sweet potato rounds with some of the scrambled eggs and the remaining sweet potato rounds. Slice the sandwiches and serve them.

Per Serving

Calorie: 222 | fat: 9g | protein: 15g | carbs: 20g | sugars: 4g | fiber: 3g | sodium: 297mg

Hoe Cakes

Prep time: 10 minutes | Cook time: 15 minutes | Makes 16 to 18

1 medium egg
½ cup fat-free milk
2 cups cornmeal
3 teaspoons baking powder

1 tablespoon unsalted non-hydrogenated plant-based butter, for greasing the pan

1. In a medium bowl, whisk the egg and milk together. 2. In a separate medium bowl, whisk the cornmeal and baking powder together. 3. Fold the dry ingredients into the wet ingredients until incorporated. 4. In a skillet, melt the butter over medium heat. 5. Add the batter in ¼-cup dollops to the pan (no more than 4 dollops at a time, spaced 1 to 2 inches apart). 6. When the edges become golden brown, turn the cakes, and cook for 30 to 60 seconds more. Repeat until no batter remains.

Per Serving

Calories: 85 | fat: 1g | protein: 2g | carbs: 16g | sugars: 1g | fiber: 1g | sodium: 10mg

Breakfast Hash

Prep time: 10 minutes | Cook time: 30 minutes | Serves 6

Oil, for spraying
3 medium russet potatoes, diced
½ yellow onion, diced
1 green bell pepper, seeded and diced

2 tablespoons olive oil
2 teaspoons granulated garlic
1 teaspoon salt
½ teaspoon freshly ground black pepper

1. Line the air fryer basket with parchment and spray lightly with oil. 2. In a large bowl, mix together the potatoes, onion, bell pepper, and olive oil. 3. Add the garlic, salt, and black pepper and stir until evenly coated. 4. Transfer the mixture to the prepared basket. 5. Air fry at 400ºF (204ºC) for 20 to 30 minutes, shaking or stirring every 10 minutes, until browned and crispy. If you spray the potatoes with a little oil each time you stir, they will get even crispier.

Per Serving

Calories: 133 | fat: 5g | protein: 3g | carbs: g21 | sugars: 2g | fiber: 2g | sodium: 395mg

Cinnamon French Toast

Prep time: 10 minutes | Cook time: 20 minutes | Serves 8

3 eggs
2 cups low-fat milk
2 tablespoons maple syrup
15 drops liquid stevia
2 teaspoons vanilla extract
2 teaspoons cinnamon

Pinch salt
16-ounces whole wheat bread, cubed and left out overnight to go stale
1½ cups water

1. In a medium bowl, whisk together the eggs, milk, maple syrup, Stevia, vanilla, cinnamon, and salt. Stir in the cubes of whole wheat bread. 2. You will need a 7-inch round baking pan for this. Spray the inside with nonstick spray, then pour the bread

mixture into the pan. 3. Place the trivet in the bottom of the inner pot, then pour in the water. 4. Make foil sling and insert it onto the trivet. Carefully place the 7-inch pan on top of the foil sling/trivet. 5. Secure the lid to the locked position, then make sure the vent is turned to sealing. 6. Press the Manual button and use the "+/-" button to set the Instant Pot for 20 minutes. 7. When cook time is up, let the Instant Pot release naturally for 5 minutes, then quick release the rest

Per Serving

Calories: 75 | fat: 3g | protein: 4g | carbs: 7g | sugars: 6g | fiber: 0g | sodium: 74mg

Hash Browns

Prep time: 5 minutes | Cook time: 10 minutes | Serves 4

2 large baking potatoes (about 10 ounces each), unpeeled
2 tablespoons minced onion
2 tablespoons minced red pepper
2 tablespoons minced green pepper

1 garlic clove, minced
½ teaspoon paprika
⅓ teaspoon salt
⅛ teaspoon freshly ground black pepper
¼ teaspoon finely chopped fresh baby dill

1. With a hand grater or a food processor with grater attachment, shred each potato. In a large bowl, combine the potatoes with the remaining ingredients. 2. Coat a large skillet with cooking spray and place over medium heat until hot. 3. Pack the potato mixture firmly into the skillet; cook for 6–8 minutes or until the bottom is browned. Invert the potato patty onto a plate and return to the skillet, cooked side up. 4. Continue cooking over medium heat for another 6–8 minutes until the bottom is browned. Remove from heat and cut into 4 wedges.

Per Serving

Calories: 89 | fat: 0g | protein: 2g | carbs: 20g | sugars: 1g | fiber: 3g | sodium: 201mg

Breakfast Casserole

Prep time: 10 minutes | Cook time: 35 minutes | Serves 12 to 15

Nonstick cooking spray
6 medium brown eggs
8 medium egg whites
1 green bell pepper, chopped
½ small yellow onion, chopped
1 zucchini, finely grated, with

water pressed out
1 cup shredded reduced-fat Cheddar cheese
1 teaspoon paprika
½ teaspoon garlic powder

1. Preheat the oven to 350°F. Spray a large cast iron skillet with cooking spray. 2. In a medium bowl, whisk the eggs and egg whites together. 3. Add the bell pepper, onion, zucchini, cheese, paprika, and garlic powder, mix well, and pour into the prepared skillet. 4. Transfer the skillet to the oven, and bake for 35 minutes. Remove from the oven, and let rest for 5 minutes before serving.

Per Serving

Calories: 66 | fat: 3g | protein: 8g | carbs: 2g | sugars: 1g | fiber: 1g | sodium: 152mg

Mandarin Orange–Millet Breakfast Bowl

Prep time: 5 minutes | Cook time: 30 minutes | Serves 2

⅓ cup millet
1 cup nonfat milk
½ cup water
¼ teaspoon cinnamon
¼ teaspoon ground cardamom
1 teaspoon vanilla extract

Pinch salt
Stevia, for sweetening
½ cup canned mandarin oranges, drained
2 tablespoons sliced almonds

1. In a small saucepan set over medium-high heat, stir together the millet, milk, water, cinnamon, cardamom, vanilla, salt, and stevia. Bring to a boil. Reduce the heat to low. Cover and simmer for 25 minutes, without stirring. If the liquid is not completely absorbed, cook for 3 to 5 minutes longer, partially covered. 2. Stir in the oranges. Remove from the heat. 3. Top with the sliced almonds and serve.

Per Serving

Calories: 254 | fat: 7g | protein: 10g | carbs: 38g | sugars: 12g | fiber: 5g | sodium: 73mg

Bran Apple Muffins

Prep time: 10 minutes | Cook time: 20 minutes | Makes 18 muffins

2 cups whole-wheat flour
1 cup wheat bran
⅓ cup granulated sweetener
1 tablespoon baking powder
2 teaspoons ground cinnamon
½ teaspoon ground ginger
¼ teaspoon ground nutmeg
Pinch sea salt

2 eggs
1½ cups skim milk, at room temperature
½ cup melted coconut oil
2 teaspoons pure vanilla extract
2 apples, peeled, cored, and diced

1. Preheat the oven to 350°F. 2. Line 18 muffin cups with paper liners and set the tray aside. 3. In a large bowl, stir together the flour, bran, sweetener, baking powder, cinnamon, ginger, nutmeg, and salt. 4. In a small bowl, whisk the eggs, milk, coconut oil, and vanilla until blended. 5. Add the wet ingredients to the dry ingredients, stirring until just blended. 6. Stir in the apples and spoon equal amounts of batter into each muffin cup. 7. Bake the muffins until a toothpick inserted in the center of a muffin comes out clean, about 20 minutes. 8. Cool the muffins completely and serve. 9. Store leftover muffins in a sealed container in the refrigerator for up to 3 days or in the freezer for up to 1 month.

Per Serving

Calories: 145 | fat: 7g | protein: 4g | carbs: 19g | sugars: 6g | fiber: 4g | sodium: 17mg

Sweet Potato Breakfast Bites

Prep time: 5 minutes | Cook time: 17 to 18 minutes | Makes 12 bites

1½ cups precooked and cooled sweet potato
½ cup pure maple syrup

1 teaspoon pure vanilla extract
1¼ cups rolled oats
1 cup oat flour

½ teaspoon cinnamon
½ teaspoon pumpkin pie spice (optional; can substitute another ½ teaspoon cinnamon)
2 teaspoons baking powder

¼ teaspoon sea salt
2–3 tablespoons raisins or sugar-free nondairy chocolate chips (optional)

1. Preheat the oven to 350°F and line a baking sheet with parchment paper. 2. In a medium bowl, mash the sweet potato. Add the syrup and vanilla and stir to combine. Add the oats, oat flour, cinnamon, pumpkin pie spice (if using), baking powder, and salt, and mix until well combined. Add the raisins or chips (if using), and stir to combine. Refrigerate for 5 to 10 minutes. Scoop 1½ tablespoon rounds of the mixture onto the parchment, spacing them 1 to 2 inches apart. Bake for 17 to 18 minutes, or until set to the touch. Remove from the oven, and let cool.

Per Serving

Calorie: 215 | fat: 2g | protein: 6g | carbs: 42g | sugars: 19g | fiber: 5g | sodium: 281mg

Savory Grits

Prep time: 5 minutes | Cook time: 7 minutes | Serves 4

2 cups water
1 cup fat-free milk

1 cup stone-ground corn grits

1. In a heavy-bottomed pot, bring the water and milk to a simmer over medium heat. 2. Gradually add the grits, stirring continuously. 3. Reduce the heat to low, cover, and cook, stirring often, for 5 to 7 minutes, or until the grits are soft and tender. Serve and enjoy.

Per Serving

Calories: 166 | fat: 1g | protein: 6g | carbs: 34g | sugars: 3g | fiber: 1g | sodium: 35mg

Veggie and Tofu Scramble

Prep time: 5 minutes | Cook time: 10 minutes | Serves 2

1 pound firm- or extra-firm tofu
1 teaspoon dry mustard
1 teaspoon ground cumin
1 tablespoon extra-virgin olive oil
2 medium tomatoes, diced
1 medium zucchini, chopped
¾ cup sliced fresh mushrooms

2 garlic cloves, minced
1 bunch spinach, rinsed and chopped
½ teaspoon low-sodium soy sauce
1 teaspoon freshly squeezed lemon juice
Freshly ground black pepper

1. In a colander, drain the tofu. 2. In a medium bowl, crumble the drained tofu. 3. Add the mustard and cumin. Toss until well mixed. 4. In a nonstick skillet set over medium-high heat, heat the olive oil. 5. Add the tomatoes, zucchini, mushrooms, and garlic. Sauté for 2 to 3 minutes. Reduce the heat to medium-low. 6. Add the spinach, tofu, soy sauce, and lemon juice. 7. Cover and cook for 5 to 7 minutes, stirring occasionally. 8. Season with pepper and serve immediately.

Per Serving

Calories: 293 | fat: 16g | protein: 23g | carbs: 21g | sugars: 9g | fiber: 7g | sodium: 239mg

Pumpkin Apple Waffles

Prep time: 10 minutes | Cook time: 20 minutes | Serves 6

2¼ cups whole-wheat pastry flour
2 tablespoons granulated sweetener
1 tablespoon baking powder
1 teaspoon ground cinnamon
1 teaspoon ground nutmeg

4 eggs
1¼ cups pure pumpkin purée
1 apple, peeled, cored, and finely chopped
Melted coconut oil, for cooking

1. In a large bowl, stir together the flour, sweetener, baking powder, cinnamon, and nutmeg. 2. In a small bowl, whisk together the eggs and pumpkin. 3. Add the wet ingredients to the dry and whisk until smooth. 4. Stir the apple into the batter. 5. Cook the waffles according to the waffle maker manufacturer's directions, brushing your waffle iron with melted coconut oil, until all the batter is gone. 6. Serve.

Per Serving

Calories: 241 | fat: 4g | protein: 10g | carbs: 44g | sugars: 7g | fiber: 7g | sodium: 46mg

Black Bean Breakfast Burrito

Prep time: 10 minutes | Cook time: 10 minutes | Serves 2

Extra-virgin olive oil cooking spray
½ cup chopped onion
½ cup chopped bell pepper, any color
1 cup canned black beans, drained and rinsed
1 cup finely chopped fresh kale, thoroughly washed

1 teaspoon ground cumin
1 teaspoon freshly squeezed lime juice
2 (7-inch) low-carb whole-wheat tortillas
½ avocado, sliced, divided
4 tablespoons salsa, divided
Shredded nonfat cheese, for garnish (optional)

1. Spray a medium skillet with cooking oil. Place it over medium-high heat. 2. Add the onion and bell pepper. Sauté for 3 minutes. 3. Add the black beans, kale, cumin, and lime juice. Stir to combine. Reduce the heat to medium-low. Cover and simmer for 5 minutes. 4. Top each tortilla with half of the avocado slices and 2 tablespoons of salsa. 5. Remove the bean mixture from the heat. Evenly divide it between the tortillas. 6. Garnish with the cheese (if using) and enjoy immediately!

Per Serving

Calories: 363 | fat: 12g | protein: 14g | carbs: 42g | sugars: 7g | fiber: 18g | sodium: 476mg

Easy Buckwheat Crêpes

Prep time: 5 minutes | Cook time: 15 minutes | Makes 12 crêpes

1 cup buckwheat flour
1¾ cups milk
⅛ teaspoon kosher salt
1 tablespoon extra-virgin olive

oil
½ tablespoon ground flaxseed (optional)

1. Combine the buckwheat flour, milk, salt, extra-virgin olive oil, and flaxseed (if using), in a bowl and whisk thoroughly, or in a blender and pulse until well combined. 2. Heat a nonstick medium skillet over medium heat. Once it's hot, add a ¼ cup of batter to the skillet, spreading it out evenly. Cook until bubbles appear and the edges crisp like a pancake, 1 to 3 minutes, then flip and cook for another 2 minutes. 3. Repeat until all the batter is used up, and the crêpes are cooked. Layer parchment paper or tea towels between the crêpes to keep them from sticking to one another while also keeping them warm until you're ready to eat. 4. Serve with the desired fillings. 5. Store any leftovers in an airtight container in the refrigerator for up to 3 days.

Per Serving1 crêpes:

Calories: 56 | fat: 2g | protein: 2g | carbs: 9g | sugars: 2g | fiber: 1g | sodium: 46mg

Goji Berry Muesli

Prep time: 30 minutes | Cook time: 0 minutes | Serves 2

½ cup old-fashioned rolled oats
½ cup plain nonfat Greek yogurt
2 tablespoons dried goji berries, or dried blueberries, cherries, or cranberries
1 teaspoon liquid stevia
½ teaspoon vanilla extract

½ cup fresh blueberries, divided
3 teaspoons pumpkin seeds, divided
3 teaspoons finely ground flaxseed, divided
½ cup unsweetened vanilla almond milk, divided

1. In a medium bowl, stir together the oats, yogurt, goji berries, stevia, and vanilla. 2. Evenly divide the mixture between 2 small bowls. Cover and refrigerate overnight. 3. The next morning, top each serving with ¼ cup of blueberries, 1½ teaspoons of pumpkin seeds, and 1½ teaspoons of flaxseed. Stir to combine. Let sit for 5 to 10 minutes. 4. Top each with ¼ cup of vanilla almond milk and enjoy cold!

Per Serving

Calories: 180 | fat: 6g | protein: 10g | carbs: 27g | sugars: 11g | fiber: 6g | sodium: 88mg

Breakfast Meatballs

Prep time: 10 minutes | Cook time: 15 minutes | Makes 18 meatballs

1 pound (454 g) ground pork breakfast sausage
½ teaspoon salt
¼ teaspoon ground black pepper

½ cup shredded sharp Cheddar cheese
1 ounce (28 g) cream cheese, softened
1 large egg, whisked

1. Combine all ingredients in a large bowl. Form mixture into eighteen 1-inch meatballs. 2. Place meatballs into ungreased air fryer basket. Adjust the temperature to 400ºF (204ºC) and air fry for 15 minutes, shaking basket three times during cooking. Meatballs will be browned on the outside and have an internal temperature of at least 145ºF (63ºC) when completely cooked. Serve warm.

Per Serving1 meatball:

Calories: 106 | fat: 9g | protein: 5g | carbs: 0g | sugars: 0g | fiber: 0g | sodium: 284mg

Cauliflower Scramble

Prep time: 5 minutes | Cook time: 5 minutes | Serves 3

1 package (12–16 ounces) medium or medium-firm tofu
3½–4 cups steamed cauliflower florets, lightly mashed
½ teaspoon onion powder
½ teaspoon garlic powder
½ teaspoon sea salt

¼ teaspoon prepared mustard
½ teaspoon black salt (or another ¼ teaspoon sea salt)
½ tablespoon tahini
2½–3 tablespoons nutritional yeast
2–3 cups chopped spinach or kale

1. In a large nonstick skillet, use your fingers to crumble the tofu, breaking it up well. Place the skillet over medium heat. Add the cauliflower, onion powder, garlic powder, sea salt, mustard, and black salt. Cook for 3 to 4 minutes, then add the tahini and nutritional yeast and stir to combine thoroughly. If the mixture is sticking, add 1 to 2 tablespoons water. Add the spinach or kale during the final minutes of cooking, stirring until just nicely wilted and still bright green. Taste, season as desired, and serve.

Per Serving

Calorie: 196 | fat: 9g | protein: 21g | carbs: 16g | sugars: 3g | fiber: 10g | sodium: 862mg

Crepe Cakes

Prep time: 5 minutes | Cook time: 20 minutes | Serves 4

Avocado oil cooking spray
4 ounces reduced-fat plain cream cheese, softened
2 medium bananas

4 large eggs
½ teaspoon vanilla extract
⅛ teaspoon salt

1. Heat a large skillet over low heat. Coat the cooking surface with cooking spray, and allow the pan to heat for another 2 to 3 minutes. 2. Meanwhile, in a medium bowl, mash the cream cheese and bananas together with a fork until combined. The bananas can be a little chunky. 3. Add the eggs, vanilla, and salt, and mix well. 4. For each cake, drop 2 tablespoons of the batter onto the warmed skillet and use the bottom of a large spoon or ladle to spread it thin. Let it cook for 7 to 9 minutes. 5. Flip the cake over and cook briefly, about 1 minute.

Per Serving

Calories: 183 | fat: 9g | protein: 9g | carbs: 16g | sugars: 9g | fiber: 2g | sodium: 251mg

Low-Carb Peanut Butter Pancakes

Prep time: 10 minutes | Cook time: 10 minutes | Serves 2

1 cup almond flour
½ teaspoon baking soda
Pinch sea salt
2 large eggs
¼ cup sparkling water (plain,

unsweetened)
2 tablespoons canola oil, plus more for cooking
4 tablespoons peanut butter

1. Heat a nonstick griddle over medium-high heat. 2. In a small bowl, whisk together the almond flour, baking soda, and salt. 3.

In a glass measuring cup, whisk together the eggs, water, and oil. 4. Pour the liquid ingredients into the dry ingredients, and mix gently until just combined. 5. Brush a small amount of canola oil onto the griddle. 6. Using all of the batter, spoon four pancakes onto the griddle. 7. Cook until set on one side, about 3 minutes. Flip with a spatula and continue cooking on the other side. 8. Before serving, spread each pancake with 1 tablespoon of the peanut butter.

Per Serving

Calories: 516 | fat: 43g | protein: 25g | carbs: 21g | sugars: 5g | fiber: 6g | sodium: 580mg

Egg Bites with Sausage and Peppers

Prep time: 5 minutes | Cook time: 15 minutes | Serves 7

4 large eggs
¼ cup vegan cream cheese (such as Tofutti brand) or cream cheese
¼ teaspoon fine sea salt
¼ teaspoon freshly ground black pepper
3 ounces lean turkey sausage, cooked and crumbled, or 1 vegetarian sausage (such as

Beyond Meat brand), cooked and diced
½ red bell pepper, seeded and chopped
2 green onions, white and green parts, minced, plus more for garnish (optional)
¼ cup vegan cheese shreds or shredded sharp Cheddar cheese

1. In a blender, combine the eggs, cream cheese, salt, and pepper. Blend on medium speed for about 20 seconds, just until combined. Add the sausage, bell pepper, and green onions and pulse for 1 second once or twice. You want to mix in the solid ingredients without grinding them up very much. 2. Pour 1 cup water into the Instant Pot. Generously grease a 7-cup egg-bite mold or seven 2-ounce silicone baking cups with butter or coconut oil, making sure to coat each cup well. Place the prepared mold or cups on a long-handled silicone steam rack. (If you don't have the long-handled rack, use the wire metal steam rack and a homemade sling) 3. Pour ¼ cup of the egg mixture into each prepared mold or cup. Holding the handles of the steam rack, carefully lower the egg bites into the pot. 4. Secure the lid and set the Pressure Release to Sealing. Select the Steam setting and set the cooking time for 8 minutes at low pressure. (The pot will take about 5 minutes to come up to pressure before the cooking program begins.) 5. When the cooking program ends, let the pressure release naturally for 5 minutes, then move the Pressure Release to Venting to release any remaining steam. Open the pot. The egg muffins will have puffed up quite a bit during cooking, but they will deflate and settle as they cool. Wearing heat-resistant mitts, grasp the handles of the steam rack and carefully lift the egg bites out of the pot. Sprinkle the egg bites with the cheese, then let them cool for about 5 minutes, until the cheese has fully melted and you are able to handle the mold or cups comfortably. 6. Pull the sides of the egg mold or cups away from the egg bites, running a butter knife around the edge of each bite to loosen if necessary. Transfer the egg bites to plates, garnish with more green onions (if desired), and serve warm. To store, let cool to room temperature, transfer to an airtight container, and refrigerate for up to 3 days; reheat gently in the microwave for about 1 minute before serving.

Per Serving

Calories: 112 | fat: 8g | protein: 8g | carbs: 3g | sugars: 0g | fiber: 0g | sodium: 297mg

Chapter 2 Vegetables and Sides

Lean Green Avocado Mashed Potatoes 20

Chipotle Twice-Baked Sweet Potatoes 20

Wild Rice Salad with Cranberries and Almonds 20

Roasted Beets, Carrots, and Parsnips 20

Asparagus with Vinaigrette 21

Roasted Delicata Squash 21

Parmesan-Rosemary Radishes 21

Chinese Asparagus 21

Broccoli Cauliflower Bake 21

Cauliflower "Mashed Potatoes" 22

Caramelized Onions 22

Spinach and Sweet Pepper Poppers 22

Lemony Brussels Sprouts with Poppy Seeds 22

Green Beans with Garlic and Onion 22

Moreish Lemony Quinoa 23

Wilted Kale and Chard 23

Garlic Roasted Broccoli 23

Sautéed Lemon Broccoli and Kale 23

Soft-Baked Tamari Tofu 23

Sherried Peppers with Bean Sprouts 23

Brussels Sprouts with Pecans and Gorgonzola 24

Pico de Gallo Navy Beans 24

Vegetable Medley 24

Parmesan Cauliflower Mash 24

Charred Miso Cabbage 24

Dijon Roast Cabbage 25

Chunky Red Pepper and Tomato Sauce 25

Garlicky Cabbage and Collard Greens 25

Sautéed Mixed Vegetables 25

Nutmeg Green Beans 25

Horseradish Mashed Cauliflower 26

Sun-Dried Tomato Brussels Sprouts 26

Zucchini on the Half Shell 26

Potatoes with Parsley 26

Green Beans with Red Peppers 26

Sweet-and-Sour Cabbage Slaw 27

Garlic Herb Radishes 27

Teriyaki Chickpeas 27

Carrots Marsala 27

Garlic Roasted Radishes 27

Ginger Broccoli 27

Cheesy Cauli Bake 28

Italian Wild Mushrooms 28

Cauliflower and Butternut Squash Mac and Cheese 28

Spicy Roasted Cauliflower with Lime 28

Lean Green Avocado Mashed Potatoes

Prep time: 15 minutes | Cook time: 30 minutes | Serves 4

2 large russet potatoes, chopped
1 large head cauliflower, cut into 1-inch (2.5-cm) florets
2 medium leeks, washed and coarsely chopped
2 teaspoons (10 ml) olive oil
1 tablespoon (3 g) dried

rosemary
1 tablespoon (3 g) dried thyme
2 cloves garlic
1 medium avocado, peeled and pitted
2 tablespoons (8 g) finely chopped fresh chives

1. Preheat the oven to 400°F (204°C). 2. Spread out the potatoes, cauliflower, and leeks on a large baking sheet. Drizzle the vegetables with the oil, then sprinkle them with the rosemary and thyme. Add the garlic to the baking sheet. Bake the vegetables for about 30 minutes, until the potatoes are fork-tender. 3. Transfer the vegetables to a food processor and add the avocado. Process the mixture to the desired consistency. 4. Top the mashed potatoes with the chives and serve.

Per Serving

Calorie: 248 | fat: 10g | protein: 7g | carbs: 37g | sugars: 6g | fiber: 9g | sodium: 69mg

Chipotle Twice-Baked Sweet Potatoes

Prep time: 20 minutes | Cook time: 1 hour | Serves 4

4 small sweet potatoes (about 1¾ pounds)
¼ cup fat-free half-and-half
1 chipotle chile in adobo sauce (from 7-ounce can), finely chopped
1 teaspoon adobo sauce (from

can of chipotle chiles)
½ teaspoon salt
8 teaspoons reduced-fat sour cream
4 teaspoons chopped fresh cilantro

1. Heat oven to 375°F. Gently scrub potatoes but do not peel. Pierce potatoes several times with fork to allow steam to escape while potatoes bake. Bake about 45 minutes or until potatoes are tender when pierced in center with a fork. 2. When potatoes are cool enough to handle, cut lengthwise down through center of potato to within ½ inch of ends and bottom. Carefully scoop out inside, leaving thin shell. In medium bowl, mash potatoes, half-and-half, chile, adobo sauce and salt with potato masher or electric mixer on low speed until light and fluffy. 3. Increase oven temperature to 400°F. In 13x9-inch pan, place potato shells. Divide potato mixture evenly among shells. Bake uncovered 20 minutes or until potato mixture is golden brown and heated through. 4. Just before serving, top each potato with 2 teaspoons sour cream and 1 teaspoon cilantro.

Per Serving

Calorie: 140 | fat: 1g | protein: 3g | carbs: 27g | sugars: 9g | fiber: 4g | sodium: 400mg

Wild Rice Salad with Cranberries and Almonds

Prep time: 10 minutes | Cook time: 25 minutes | Serves 18

For the rice
2 cups wild rice blend, rinsed
1 teaspoon kosher salt
2½ cups Vegetable Broth or Chicken Bone Broth
For the dressing
¼ cup extra-virgin olive oil
¼ cup white wine vinegar
1½ teaspoons grated orange zest

Juice of 1 medium orange (about ¼ cup)
1 teaspoon honey or pure maple syrup
For the salad
¾ cup unsweetened dried cranberries
½ cup sliced almonds, toasted
Freshly ground black pepper

Make the Rice 1. In the electric pressure cooker, combine the rice, salt, and broth. 2. Close and lock the lid. Set the valve to sealing. 3. Cook on high pressure for 25 minutes. 4. When the cooking is complete, hit Cancel and allow the pressure to release naturally for 15 minutes, then quick release any remaining pressure. 5. Once the pin drops, unlock and remove the lid. 6. Let the rice cool briefly, then fluff it with a fork. Make the Dressing 7. While the rice cooks, make the dressing: In a small jar with a screw-top lid, combine the olive oil, vinegar, zest, juice, and honey. (If you don't have a jar, whisk the ingredients together in a small bowl.) Shake to combine. Make the Salad 8. In a large bowl, combine the rice, cranberries, and almonds. 9. Add the dressing and season with pepper. 10. Serve warm or refrigerate.

Per Serving

Calories: 129 | fat: 4.25g | protein: 3.46g | carbs: 20.34g | sugars: 5.08g | fiber: 1.7g | sodium: 200mg

Roasted Beets, Carrots, and Parsnips

Prep time: 10 minutes | Cook time: 30 minutes | Serves 4

1 pound beets, peeled and quartered
½ pound carrots, peeled and cut into chunks
½ pound parsnips, peeled and cut into chunks

1 tablespoon extra-virgin olive oil
1 teaspoon apple cider vinegar
Sea salt
Freshly ground black pepper

1. Preheat the oven to 375°F. Line a baking tray with aluminum foil. 2. In a large bowl, toss the beets, carrots, and parsnips with the oil and vinegar until everything is well coated. Spread them out on the baking sheet. 3. Roast until the vegetables are tender and lightly caramelized, about 30 minutes. 4. Transfer the vegetables to a serving bowl, season with salt and pepper, and serve warm.

Per Serving

Calories: 122 | fat: 3.84g | protein: 3.73g | carbs: 20.75g | sugars: 5.98g | fiber: 8.6g | sodium: 592mg

Asparagus with Vinaigrette

Prep time: 5 minutes | Cook time: 10 minutes | Serves 6

1½ pounds fresh or frozen asparagus (thin pieces)
½ cup red wine vinegar
½ teaspoon dried or 1 teaspoon fresh tarragon
2 tablespoons finely chopped fresh chives
3 tablespoons finely chopped fresh parsley
½ cup water
1 tablespoon extra-virgin olive oil
1⅓ tablespoons Dijon mustard
1 pound fresh spinach leaves, trimmed of stems, washed, and dried
2 large tomatoes, cut into wedges

1. Place 1 inch of water in a pot, and place a steamer inside. Arrange the asparagus on top of the steamer. Steam fresh asparagus for 4 minutes or frozen asparagus for 6–8 minutes. Immediately rinse the asparagus under cold water to stop the cooking. (This helps keep asparagus bright green and crunchy.) Set aside. 2. In a small bowl or salad cruet, combine the remaining ingredients except the spinach and tomatoes. Mix, or shake well. 3. To serve, line plates with the spinach leaves, and place the asparagus on top of the spinach. Garnish with the tomato wedges, and spoon any remaining dressing on top.

Per Serving

Calories: 72 | fat: 1.82g | protein: 6.61g | carbs: 10.2g | sugars: 1.98g | fiber: 4.8g | sodium: 133mg

Roasted Delicata Squash

Prep time: 10 minutes | Cook time: 20 minutes | Serves 4

1 (1- to 1½-pound) delicata squash, halved, seeded, cut into ½-inch-thick strips
1 tablespoon extra-virgin olive oil
½ teaspoon dried thyme
¼ teaspoon salt
¼ teaspoon freshly ground black pepper

1. Preheat the oven to 400°F. Line a baking sheet with parchment paper. 2. In a large mixing bowl, toss the squash strips with the olive oil, thyme, salt, and pepper. Arrange on the prepared baking sheet in a single layer. 3. Roast for 10 minutes, flip, and continue to roast for 10 more minutes until tender and lightly browned.

Per Serving

Calories: 79 | fat: 4g | protein: 1g | carbs: 12g | sugars: 3g | fiber: 2g | sodium: 123mg

Parmesan-Rosemary Radishes

Prep time: 5 minutes | Cook time: 15 to 20 minutes | Serves 4

1 bunch radishes, stemmed, trimmed, and quartered
1 tablespoon avocado oil
2 tablespoons finely grated fresh Parmesan cheese
1 tablespoon chopped fresh rosemary
Sea salt and freshly ground black pepper, to taste

1. Place the radishes in a medium bowl and toss them with the avocado oil, Parmesan cheese, rosemary, salt, and pepper. 2. Set the air fryer to 375°F (191°C). Arrange the radishes in a single layer in the air fryer basket. Roast for 15 to 20 minutes, until golden brown and tender. Let cool for 5 minutes before serving.

Per Serving

Calories: 58 | fat: 4.32g | protein: 1.26g | carbs: 4.09g | sugars: 2.12g | fiber: 1.5g | sodium: 63mg

Chinese Asparagus

Prep time: 5 minutes | Cook time: 5 minutes | Serves 4

1 pound asparagus
½ cup plus 1 tablespoon water, divided
1 tablespoon light soy sauce
1 tablespoon rice vinegar
2 teaspoons cornstarch
1 tablespoon canola oil
2 teaspoons grated fresh ginger
1 scallion, minced

1. Trim the tough ends off the asparagus. Cut the stalks diagonally into 2-inch pieces. 2. In a small bowl, combine the ½ cup water, soy sauce, and rice vinegar. 3. In a measuring cup, combine the cornstarch and 1 tablespoon water. Set aside. 4. Heat the oil in a wok or skillet. Add the ginger and scallions, and stir-fry for 30 seconds. Add the asparagus and stir-fry for a few seconds more. Add the broth mixture, and bring to a boil. Cover, and simmer for 3–5 minutes, until the asparagus is just tender. 5. Add the cornstarch mixture, and cook until thickened. Serve.

Per Serving

Calories: 73 | fat: 4.37g | protein: 2.87g | carbs: 7.09g | sugars: 3.02g | fiber: 2.6g | sodium: 64mg

Broccoli Cauliflower Bake

Prep time: 15 minutes | Cook time: 40 minutes | Serves 6

½ cup ground almonds
¼ cup grated Parmesan cheese
1 tablespoon butter, melted, plus 2 tablespoons butter
Pinch freshly ground black pepper
1 head broccoli, cut into small florets
1 head cauliflower, cut into small florets
1 sweet onion, chopped
1 teaspoon minced garlic
2 tablespoons all-purpose flour
1 cup skim milk
2 ounces goat cheese
¼ teaspoon ground nutmeg

1. Preheat the oven to 350°F. 2. In a small bowl, mix together the almonds, Parmesan cheese, melted butter, and pepper. Set it aside. 3. Place a large pot full of water over high heat and bring to a boil. 4. Blanch the broccoli and cauliflower for 1 minute, drain, and set them aside. 5. Place a large skillet over medium-high heat and melt the 2 tablespoons of butter. 6. Sauté the onion and garlic until tender, about 3 minutes. Whisk in the flour and cook, stirring constantly, for 1 minute. Whisk in the milk and cook, stirring constantly, until the sauce has thickened, about 4 minutes. 7. Remove the skillet from the heat and whisk in the goat cheese and nutmeg. 8. Add the broccoli and cauliflower, then spoon the mixture into a 1½-quart casserole dish. 9. Sprinkle the almond mixture over the top and bake until the casserole is heated through, about 30 minutes.

Per Serving

Calories: 212 | fat: 8g | protein: 13g | carbs: 27g | sugars: 10g | fiber: 7g | sodium: 241mg

Cauliflower "Mashed Potatoes"

Prep time: 5 minutes | Cook time: 0 minutes | Serves 2

2 cups cooked cauliflower florets
1 tablespoon plain nonfat Greek yogurt
½ teaspoon extra-virgin olive

oil
Salt, to season
Freshly ground black pepper, to season

1. To a food processor, add the cauliflower, yogurt, and olive oil. Process until smooth. 2. Season with salt and pepper before serving.

Per Serving

Calories: 50 | fat: 1.8g | protein: 3.93g | carbs: 6.37g | sugars: 3.07g | fiber: 3.1g | sodium: 606mg

Caramelized Onions

Prep time: 10 minutes | Cook time: 35 minutes | Serves 8

4 tablespoons margarine
6 large Vidalia or other sweet onions, sliced into thin half

rings
10-ounce can chicken, or vegetable, broth

1. Press Sauté on the Instant Pot. Add in the margarine and let melt. 2. Once the margarine is melted, stir in the onions and sauté for about 5 minutes. Pour in the broth and then press Cancel. 3. Secure the lid and make sure vent is set to sealing. Press Manual and set time for 20 minutes. 4. When cook time is up, release the pressure manually. Remove the lid and press Sauté. Stir the onion mixture for about 10 more minutes, allowing extra liquid to cook off.

Per Serving

Calorie: 123 | fat: 6g | protein: 2g | carbs: 15g | sugars: 10g | fiber: 3g | sodium: 325mg

Spinach and Sweet Pepper Poppers

Prep time: 10 minutes | Cook time: 8 minutes | Makes 16 poppers

4 ounces (113 g) cream cheese, softened
1 cup chopped fresh spinach leaves

½ teaspoon garlic powder
8 mini sweet bell peppers, tops removed, seeded, and halved lengthwise

1. In a medium bowl, mix cream cheese, spinach, and garlic powder. Place 1 tablespoon mixture into each sweet pepper half and press down to smooth. 2. Place poppers into ungreased air fryer basket. Adjust the temperature to 400ºF (204ºC) and air fry for 8 minutes. Poppers will be done when cheese is browned on top and peppers are tender-crisp. Serve warm.

Per Serving

Calories: 31 | fat: 2.08g | protein: 1.02g | carbs: 2.52g | sugars: 1.41g | fiber: 0.4g | sodium: 34mg

Lemony Brussels Sprouts with Poppy Seeds

Prep time: 10 minutes | Cook time: 2 minutes | Serves 4

1 pound (454 g) Brussels sprouts
2 tablespoons avocado oil, divided
1 cup vegetable broth or chicken bone broth

1 tablespoon minced garlic
½ teaspoon kosher salt
Freshly ground black pepper, to taste
½ medium lemon
½ tablespoon poppy seeds

1. Trim the Brussels sprouts by cutting off the stem ends and removing any loose outer leaves. Cut each in half lengthwise (through the stem). 2. Set the electric pressure cooker to the Sauté/More setting. When the pot is hot, pour in 1 tablespoon of the avocado oil. 3. Add half of the Brussels sprouts to the pot, cut-side down, and let them brown for 3 to 5 minutes without disturbing. Transfer to a bowl and add the remaining tablespoon of avocado oil and the remaining Brussels sprouts to the pot. Hit Cancel and return all of the Brussels sprouts to the pot. 4. Add the broth, garlic, salt, and a few grinds of pepper. Stir to distribute the seasonings. 5. Close and lock the lid of the pressure cooker. Set the valve to sealing. 6. Cook on high pressure for 2 minutes. 7. While the Brussels sprouts are cooking, zest the lemon, then cut it into quarters. 8. When the cooking is complete, hit Cancel and quick release the pressure. 9. Once the pin drops, unlock and remove the lid. 10. Using a slotted spoon, transfer the Brussels sprouts to a serving bowl. Toss with the lemon zest, a squeeze of lemon juice, and the poppy seeds. Serve immediately.

Per Serving

Calories: 125 | fat: 8g | protein: 4g | carbs: 13g | sugars: 3g | fiber: 5g | sodium: 504mg

Green Beans with Garlic and Onion

Prep time: 5 minutes | Cook time: 12 minutes | Serves 8

1 pound fresh green beans, trimmed and cut into 2-inch pieces
1 tablespoon extra-virgin olive oil
1 small onion, chopped

1 large garlic clove, minced
1 tablespoon white vinegar
¼ cup Parmigiano-Reggiano cheese
⅛ teaspoon freshly ground black pepper

1. Steam the beans for 7 minutes or until just tender. Set aside. 2. In a skillet, heat the oil over low heat. Add the onion and garlic, and sauté for 4–5 minutes or until the onion is translucent. 3. Transfer the beans to a serving bowl, and add the onion mixture and vinegar, tossing well. Sprinkle with cheese and pepper, and serve.

Per Serving

Calories: 43 | fat: 2.87g | protein: 1.45g | carbs: 3.55g | sugars: 0.91g | fiber: 1.2g | sodium: 30mg

Moreish Lemony Quinoa

Prep time: 5 minutes | Cook time: 15 minutes | Serves 3

1 cup dry quinoa, rinsed and drained
1¾ cups water
2½ tablespoons tamari
2 tablespoons tahini
3–4 tablespoons fresh lemon juice
½ teaspoon garlic powder

1. In a large saucepan over high heat, combine the quinoa and water. Bring to a boil, stir, then reduce the heat to low. Cover and cook for 11 minutes. In a small bowl, combine the tamari, tahini, lemon juice, and garlic powder. Whisk to combine. Once the quinoa is cooked, turn off the heat and stir in the tahini mixture. Cover again, let sit for a couple of minutes, and serve.

Per Serving

Calorie: 281 | fat: 9g | protein: 11g | carbs: 40g | sugars: 4g | fiber: 5g | sodium: 861mg

Wilted Kale and Chard

Prep time: 10 minutes | Cook time: 10 minutes | Serves 4

2 tablespoons extra-virgin olive oil
1 pound kale, coarse stems removed and leaves chopped
1 pound Swiss chard, coarse stems removed and leaves
chopped
1 tablespoon freshly squeezed lemon juice
½ teaspoon ground cardamom
Sea salt
Freshly ground black pepper

1. Place a large skillet over medium-high heat and add the olive oil. 2. Add the kale, chard, lemon juice, and cardamom to the skillet. Use tongs to toss the greens continuously until they are wilted, about 10 minutes or less. 3. Season the greens with salt and pepper. 4. Serve immediately.

Per Serving

Calories: 139 | fat: 8.06g | protein: 6.95g | carbs: 14.69g | sugars: 3.91g | fiber: 6g | sodium: 430mg

Garlic Roasted Broccoli

Prep time: 8 minutes | Cook time: 10 to 14 minutes | Serves 6

1 head broccoli, cut into bite-size florets
1 tablespoon avocado oil
2 teaspoons minced garlic
⅛ teaspoon red pepper flakes
Sea salt and freshly ground black pepper, to taste
1 tablespoon freshly squeezed lemon juice
½ teaspoon lemon zest

1. In a large bowl, toss together the broccoli, avocado oil, garlic, red pepper flakes, salt, and pepper. 2. Set the air fryer to 375°F (191°C). Arrange the broccoli in a single layer in the air fryer basket, working in batches if necessary. Roast for 10 to 14 minutes, until the broccoli is lightly charred. 3. Place the florets in a medium bowl and toss with the lemon juice and lemon zest. Serve.

Per Serving

Calories: 58 | fat: 2.73g | protein: 2.95g | carbs: 7.37g | sugars: 1.81g | fiber: 2.7g | sodium: 34mg

Sautéed Lemon Broccoli and Kale

Prep time: 5 minutes | Cook time: 15 minutes | Serves 4 to 6

1 large head broccoli, cut into small florets
2 tablespoons extra-virgin olive oil
1 bunch kale, torn into 1- to
2-inch pieces
2 garlic cloves, minced
½ teaspoon cumin seeds
1 lemon, cut into wedges

1. Bring a medium saucepan filled three-quarters full of water to a boil over high heat. Add the broccoli and boil for 3 minutes. Drain the broccoli and run it under cold water until completely cool. 2. Heat the extra-virgin olive oil in a large skillet over medium-high heat. Add the broccoli, kale, garlic, and cumin and sauté for 2 to 3 minutes. Remove the skillet from the heat and serve with freshly squeezed lemon. 3. Store any leftovers in an airtight container in the refrigerator for 3 to 4 days.

Per Serving

Calories: 122 | fat: 5.43g | protein: 6.63g | carbs: 16.26g | sugars: 4.13g | fiber: 6.1g | sodium: 77mg

Soft-Baked Tamari Tofu

Prep time: 5 minutes | Cook time: 20 to 25 minutes | Serves 4

3 tablespoons tamari
1 package (16 ounces)
medium-firm tofu

1. Preheat the oven to 425°F. In an ovenproof dish just large enough to hold the tofu, add about half of the tamari. Use several paper towels to pat or squeeze some of the excess moisture from the tofu. Add the tofu to the dish, breaking it up slightly. Sprinkle the remaining tamari over the tofu. Bake for 20 to 25 minutes, or until the tofu is browned and drying in spots. Serve, spooning out tofu with some of the remaining tamari.

Per Serving

Calorie: 87 | fat: 5g | protein: 10g | carbs: 3g | sugars: 1g | fiber: 1g | sodium: 768mg

Sherried Peppers with Bean Sprouts

Prep time: 5 minutes | Cook time: 8 minutes | Serves 4

1 green bell pepper, julienned
1 red bell pepper, julienned
2 cups canned, drained bean sprouts
2 teaspoons light soy sauce
1 tablespoon dry sherry
1 teaspoon red wine vinegar

1. In a large skillet over medium heat, combine the peppers, bean sprouts, soy sauce, and sherry, mixing well. Cover, and cook 5–7 minutes, until the vegetables are just tender. 2. Stir in the vinegar, and remove from the heat. Serve hot.

Per Serving

Calories: 34 | fat: 0.66g | protein: 1.63g | carbs: 6.07g | sugars: 4.09g | fiber: 1.8g | sodium: 131mg

Brussels Sprouts with Pecans and Gorgonzola

Prep time: 10 minutes | Cook time: 25 minutes | Serves 4

½ cup pecans
1½ pounds (680 g) fresh Brussels sprouts, trimmed and quartered
2 tablespoons olive oil

Salt and freshly ground black pepper, to taste
¼ cup crumbled Gorgonzola cheese

1. Spread the pecans in a single layer of the air fryer and set the heat to 350ºF (177ºC). Air fry for 3 to 5 minutes until the pecans are lightly browned and fragrant. Transfer the pecans to a plate and continue preheating the air fryer, increasing the heat to 400ºF (204ºC). 2. In a large bowl, toss the Brussels sprouts with the olive oil and season with salt and black pepper to taste. 3. Working in batches if necessary, arrange the Brussels sprouts in a single layer in the air fryer basket. Pausing halfway through the baking time to shake the basket, air fry for 20 to 25 minutes until the sprouts are tender and starting to brown on the edges. 4. Transfer the sprouts to a serving bowl and top with the toasted pecans and Gorgonzola. Serve warm or at room temperature.

Per Serving

Calories: 253 | fat: 18.97g | protein: 8.9g | carbs: 17.24g | sugars: 4.26g | fiber: 7.7g | sodium: 96mg

Pico de Gallo Navy Beans

Prep time: 20 minutes | Cook time: 0 minutes | Serves 4

2½ cups cooked navy beans
1 tomato, diced
½ red bell pepper, seeded and chopped
¼ jalapeño pepper, chopped
1 scallion, white and green

parts, chopped
1 teaspoon minced garlic
1 teaspoon ground cumin
½ teaspoon ground coriander
½ cup low-sodium feta cheese

1. Put the beans, tomato, bell pepper, jalapeño, scallion, garlic, cumin, and coriander in a medium bowl and stir until well mixed. 2. Top with the feta cheese and serve.

Per Serving

Calories: 218 | fat: 3.74g | protein: 14.49g | carbs: 32.63g | sugars: 1.87g | fiber: 12.6g | sodium: 6mg

Vegetable Medley

Prep time: 20 minutes | Cook time: 2 minutes | Serves 8

2 medium parsnips
4 medium carrots
1 turnip, about 4½ inches diameter
1 cup water

1 teaspoon salt
3 tablespoons sugar
2 tablespoons canola or olive oil
½ teaspoon salt

1. Clean and peel vegetables. Cut in 1-inch pieces. 2. Place the cup of water and 1 teaspoon salt into the Instant Pot's inner pot with the vegetables. 3. Secure the lid and make sure vent is set to sealing. Press Manual and set for 2 minutes. 4. When cook time is up, release the pressure manually and press Cancel. Drain the water from the inner pot. 5. Press Sauté and stir in sugar, oil, and salt. Cook until sugar is dissolved. Serve.

Per Serving

Calories: 63 | fat: 2g | protein: 1g | carbs: 12g | sugars: 6g | fiber: 2g | sodium: 327mg

Parmesan Cauliflower Mash

Prep time: 7 minutes | Cook time: 5 minutes | Serves 4

1 head cauliflower, cored and cut into large florets
½ teaspoon kosher salt
½ teaspoon garlic pepper
2 tablespoons plain Greek yogurt

¾ cup freshly grated Parmesan cheese
1 tablespoon unsalted butter or ghee (optional)
Chopped fresh chives

1. Pour 1 cup of water into the electric pressure cooker and insert a steamer basket or wire rack. 2. Place the cauliflower in the basket. 3. Close and lock the lid of the pressure cooker. Set the valve to sealing. 4. Cook on high pressure for 5 minutes. 5. When the cooking is complete, hit Cancel and quick release the pressure. 6. Once the pin drops, unlock and remove the lid. 7. Remove the cauliflower from the pot and pour out the water. Return the cauliflower to the pot and add the salt, garlic pepper, yogurt, and cheese. Use an immersion blender or potato masher to purée or mash the cauliflower in the pot. 8. Spoon into a serving bowl, and garnish with butter (if using) and chives.

Per Serving

Calories: 141 | fat: 6g | protein: 12g | carbs: 12g | sugars: 9g | fiber: 4g | sodium: 592mg

Charred Miso Cabbage

Prep time: 5 minutes | Cook time: 20 minutes | Serves 4

3 tablespoons avocado oil
1 head green cabbage, cut into 8 wedges
3 tablespoons yellow or white

miso
2 tablespoons rice wine vinegar
1 lime, cut into 8 wedges

1. Preheat the oven to 400°F. Line a baking sheet with parchment paper. 2. Heat the avocado oil in a large cast-iron pan or skillet over high heat. Arrange 2 or 3 cabbage wedges in the skillet and cook for about 3 minutes on each side until charred or lightly blackened. When they're seared on both sides, place the wedges on the baking sheet. 3. Repeat with the remaining wedges. 4. In a small bowl, mix the miso with the rice wine vinegar and brush it on the cabbage wedges evenly. Bake the wedges for 10 minutes. 5. When the wedges come out of the oven, squeeze the lime juice on them. Serve. 6. Store any leftovers in an airtight container in the refrigerator for 2 to 3 days.

Per Serving

Calories: 125 | fat: 11.38g | protein: 1.61g | carbs: 4.61g | sugars: 1.12g | fiber: 0.8g | sodium: 491mg

Dijon Roast Cabbage

Prep time: 10 minutes | Cook time: 10 minutes | Serves 4

1 small head cabbage, cored and sliced into 1-inch-thick slices
2 tablespoons olive oil, divided
½ teaspoon salt
1 tablespoon Dijon mustard
1 teaspoon apple cider vinegar
1 teaspoon granular erythritol

1. Drizzle each cabbage slice with 1 tablespoon olive oil, then sprinkle with salt. Place slices into ungreased air fryer basket, working in batches if needed. Adjust the temperature to 350°F (177°C) and air fry for 10 minutes. Cabbage will be tender and edges will begin to brown when done. 2. In a small bowl, whisk remaining olive oil with mustard, vinegar, and erythritol. Drizzle over cabbage in a large serving dish. Serve warm.

Per Serving

Calories: 110 | fat: 7.34g | protein: 2.5g | carbs: 10.74g | sugars: 5.47g | fiber: 3.1g | sodium: 392mg

Chunky Red Pepper and Tomato Sauce

Prep time: 5 minutes | Cook time: 40 minutes | Makes 2½ cups

3 large red bell peppers, halved lengthwise, seeded, pressed open to flatten
2 tablespoons extra-virgin olive oil, plus additional for brushing the peppers
1 medium onion, minced
1½ teaspoons dried basil
1 teaspoon dried rosemary
½ teaspoon dried oregano
½ teaspoon salt
½ cup low-sodium vegetable broth
2 cups water
½ cup tomato purée
1 tablespoon tomato paste
2 teaspoons white wine vinegar
2 tablespoons chopped fresh basil leaves

1. Preheat the broiler to high. 2. Brush the red bell peppers with olive oil. Place them under the broiler, skin-side up. Cook for about 10 minutes, or until lightly charred. Transfer the peppers to a cutting board, stacking one on top of the other to create steam. Let sit for 10 minutes. Remove as much charred skin as possible. Slice into strips. 3. In a large skillet set over medium-high heat, heat the remaining 2 tablespoons of olive oil. 4. Add the red pepper strips, onion, basil, rosemary, oregano, and salt. Cook for 5 minutes, stirring. 5. Add the vegetable broth. Cook for about 15 minutes more, or until the mixture reduces to a sauce. 6. Add the water, tomato purée, and tomato paste. Reduce the heat to low. Simmer for 25 minutes. 7. Transfer the mixture to a food processor. Purée until smooth, but with some texture remaining. 8. Place the skillet back over low heat. Return the sauce to the skillet. Barely simmer for 1 to 2 minutes to rewarm. Stir in the white wine vinegar and basil. Serve warm. 9. Refrigerate any remaining sauce. Serve chilled or rewarmed, as desired.

Per Serving

Calories: 246 | fat: 14.67g | protein: 4.47g | carbs: 25.9g | sugars: 16.42g | fiber: 7.6g | sodium: 641mg

Garlicky Cabbage and Collard Greens

Prep time: 10 minutes | Cook time: 10 minutes | Serves 8

2 tablespoons extra-virgin olive oil
1 collard greens bunch, stemmed and thinly sliced
½ small green cabbage, thinly sliced
6 garlic cloves, minced
1 tablespoon low-sodium gluten-free soy sauce or tamari

1. In a large skillet, heat the oil over medium-high heat. 2. Add the collards to the pan, stirring to coat with oil. Sauté for 1 to 2 minutes until the greens begin to wilt. 3. Add the cabbage and stir to coat. Cover and reduce the heat to medium low. Continue to cook for 5 to 7 minutes, stirring once or twice, until the greens are tender. 4. Add the garlic and soy sauce and stir to incorporate. Cook until just fragrant, about 30 seconds longer. Serve warm and enjoy!

Per Serving

Calories: 72| fat: 4g | protein: 3g | carbs: 6g | sugars: 0g | fiber: 3g | sodium: 129mg

Sautéed Mixed Vegetables

Prep time: 20 minutes | Cook time: 8 minutes | Serves 4

2 teaspoons extra-virgin olive oil
2 carrots, peeled and sliced
4 cups broccoli florets
4 cups cauliflower florets
1 red bell pepper, seeded and cut into long strips
1 cup green beans, trimmed
Sea salt
Freshly ground black pepper

1. Place a large skillet over medium heat and add the olive oil. 2. Sauté the carrots, broccoli, and cauliflower until tender-crisp, about 6 minutes. 3. Add the bell pepper and green beans, and sauté 2 minutes more. 4. Season with salt and pepper, and serve.

Per Serving

Calories: 97 | fat: 3.16g | protein: 5.39g | carbs: 15.14g | sugars: 5.21g | fiber: 6g | sodium: 211mg

Nutmeg Green Beans

Prep time: 15 minutes | Cook time: 5 minutes | Serves 12

1 tablespoon butter
1½ pounds green beans, trimmed
1 teaspoon ground nutmeg
Sea salt

1. Place a large skillet over medium heat and melt the butter. 2. Add the green beans and sauté, stirring often, until the beans are tender-crisp, about 5 minutes. 3. Stir in the nutmeg and season with salt. 4. Serve immediately.

Per Serving

Calories: 22 | fat: 1.29g | protein: 0.66g | carbs: 2.54 g | sugars: 0.45g | fiber: 1.1g | sodium: 57mg

Horseradish Mashed Cauliflower

Prep time: 5 minutes | Cook time: 10 minutes | Serves 4

1 large head cauliflower (about 3 pounds), cut into small florets
½ cup skim milk
2 tablespoons prepared

horseradish
¼ teaspoon sea salt
2 teaspoons chopped fresh chives

1. Place a large pot of water on high heat and bring it to a boil. 2. Blanch the cauliflower until it is tender, about 5 minutes. 3. Drain the cauliflower completely and transfer it to a food processor. 4. Add the milk and horseradish to the cauliflower and purée until it is smooth and thick, about 2 minutes. Or mash it by hand with a potato masher. 5. Transfer the mashed cauliflower to a bowl and season with salt. 6. Serve immediately, topped with the chopped chives.

Per Serving

Calories: 102 | fat: 1g | protein: 8g | carbs: 19g | sugars: 9g | fiber: 7g | sodium: 292mg

Sun-Dried Tomato Brussels Sprouts

Prep time: 15 minutes | Cook time: 20 minutes | Serves 4

1 pound Brussels sprouts, trimmed and halved
1 tablespoon extra-virgin olive oil
Sea salt
Freshly ground black pepper

½ cup sun-dried tomatoes, chopped
2 tablespoons freshly squeezed lemon juice
1 teaspoon lemon zest

1. Preheat the oven to 400°F. Line a large baking sheet with aluminum foil. 2. In a large bowl, toss the Brussels sprouts with oil and season with salt and pepper. 3. Spread the Brussels sprouts on the baking sheet in a single layer. 4. Roast the sprouts until they are caramelized, about 20 minutes. 5. Transfer the sprouts to a serving bowl. Mix in the sun-dried tomatoes, lemon juice, and lemon zest. 6. Stir to combine, and serve.

Per Serving

Calories: 98 | fat: 3.94g | protein: 4.83g | carbs: 14.62g | sugars: 5.26g | fiber: 5.2g | sodium: 191mg

Zucchini on the Half Shell

Prep time: 15 minutes | Cook time: 30 minutes | Serves 4 to 8

4 zucchini, cut lengthwise, seeded, pulp removed
1 (13.4-ounce) box borlotti beans, rinsed
½ onion, finely chopped
1 garlic clove, minced

1 cup coarsely chopped tomatoes
2 teaspoons Creole seasoning
½ cup grated reduced-fat Cheddar cheese

1. Preheat the oven to 350°F. 2. Arrange the zucchini on a rimmed baking sheet in a single layer, cavity-side up. 3. Transfer the baking sheet to the oven, and bake for 10 minutes, or until the exterior of the zucchini is soft. 4. Meanwhile, in a small pan, combine the beans, onion, garlic, tomatoes, and Creole seasoning. Cook over medium heat, stirring often, for 3 to 5 minutes, or until the onion and garlic are translucent. Remove from the heat. 5. Remove the zucchini from the oven, and spoon the tomato and bean mixture into the cavities. 6. Sprinkle 1 tablespoon of cheese on top of each stuffed zucchini. 7. Return the baking sheet to the oven and cook for 10 to 15 minutes, or until the cheese is melted and golden brown. Serve warm and enjoy.

Per Serving

Calories: 63 | fat: 1.45g | protein: 5.13g | carbs: 8.66g | sugars: 4.81g | fiber: 2.7g | sodium: 177mg

Potatoes with Parsley

Prep time: 10 minutes | Cook time: 5 minutes | Serves 4

3 tablespoons margarine, divided
2 pounds medium red potatoes (about 2 ounces each), halved lengthwise
1 clove garlic, minced

½ teaspoon salt
½ cup low-sodium chicken broth
2 tablespoons chopped fresh parsley

1. Place 1 tablespoon margarine in the inner pot of the Instant Pot and select Sauté. 2. After margarine is melted, add potatoes, garlic, and salt, stirring well. 3. Sauté 4 minutes, stirring frequently. 4. Add chicken broth and stir well. 5. Seal lid, make sure vent is on sealing, then select Manual for 5 minutes on high pressure. 6. When cooking time is up, manually release the pressure. 7. Strain potatoes, toss with remaining 2 tablespoons margarine and chopped parsley, and serve immediately.

Per Serving

Calories: 237 | fat: 9g | protein: 5g | carbs: 37g | sugars: 3g | fiber: 4g | sodium: 389mg

Green Beans with Red Peppers

Prep time: 5 minutes | Cook time: 15 minutes | Serves 2

8 ounces fresh green beans, broken into 2-inch pieces
6 sun-dried tomatoes (not packed in oil), halved
1 medium red bell pepper, cut into ¼-inch strips

1 teaspoon extra-virgin olive oil
Salt, to season
Freshly ground black pepper, to season

1. In a 1-quart saucepan set over high heat, add the green beans to 1 inch of water. Bring to a boil. Boil for 5 minutes, uncovered. 2. Add the sun-dried tomatoes. Cover and boil 5 to 7 minutes more, or until the beans are crisp-tender, and the tomatoes have softened. Drain. Transfer to a serving bowl. 3. Add the red bell pepper and olive oil. Season with salt and pepper. Toss to coat. 4. Serve warm.

Per Serving

Calories: 82 | fat: 3.17g | protein: 2.83g | carbs: 12.57g | sugars: 5.65g | fiber: 4.4g | sodium: 601mg

Sweet-and-Sour Cabbage Slaw

Prep time: 10 minutes | Cook time: 0 minutes | Serves 2

2 tablespoons apple cider vinegar
1 tablespoon granulated stevia
2 cups angel hair cabbage

1 tart apple, cored and diced
½ cup shredded carrot
2 medium scallions, sliced
2 tablespoons sliced almonds

1. In a medium bowl, stir together the vinegar and stevia. 2. In a large bowl, mix together the cabbage, apple, carrot, and scallions. 3. Pour the sweetened vinegar over the vegetable mixture. Toss to combine. 4. Garnish with the sliced almonds and serve.

Per Serving

Calories: 125 | fat: 0.99g | protein: 2.29g | carbs: 29.51g | sugars: 20.87g | fiber: 5.4g | sodium: 47mg

Garlic Herb Radishes

Prep time: 10 minutes | Cook time: 10 minutes | Serves 4

1 pound (454 g) radishes
2 tablespoons unsalted butter, melted
½ teaspoon garlic powder

½ teaspoon dried parsley
¼ teaspoon dried oregano
¼ teaspoon ground black pepper

1. Remove roots from radishes and cut into quarters. 2. In a small bowl, add butter and seasonings. Toss the radishes in the herb butter and place into the air fryer basket. 3. Adjust the temperature to 350ºF (177ºC) and set the timer for 10 minutes. 4. Halfway through the cooking time, toss the radishes in the air fryer basket. Continue cooking until edges begin to turn brown. 5. Serve warm.

Per Serving

Calories: 57 | fat: 3.98g | protein: 1.01g | carbs: 5.11g | sugars: 2.85g | fiber: 1.9g | sodium: 27mg

Teriyaki Chickpeas

Prep time: 5 minutes | Cook time: 20 to 25 minutes | Serves 7

2 cans (15 ounces each) chickpeas, rinsed and drained
1½ tablespoons tamari
1 tablespoon pure maple syrup
1 tablespoon lemon juice

½–¾ teaspoon garlic powder
½ teaspoon ground ginger
½ teaspoon blackstrap molasses

1. Preheat the oven to 450°F. Line a baking sheet with parchment paper. 2. In a large mixing bowl, combine the chickpeas, tamari, syrup, lemon juice, garlic powder, ginger, and molasses. Toss to combine. Spread evenly on the prepared baking sheet and bake for 20 to 25 minutes, or until the marinade is absorbed. Serve warm, or refrigerate to enjoy later.

Per Serving

Calorie: 120 | fat: 2 | protein: 6g | carbs: 20g | sugars: 5g | fiber: 5g | sodium: 382mg

Carrots Marsala

Prep time: 5 minutes | Cook time: 10 minutes | Serves 6

10 carrots (about 1 pound), peeled and diagonally sliced
¼ cup Marsala wine
¼ cup water
1 tablespoon extra-virgin olive

oil
⅛ teaspoon freshly ground black pepper
1 tablespoon finely chopped fresh parsley

1. In a large saucepan, combine the carrots, wine, water, oil, and pepper. Bring to a boil, cover, reduce the heat, and simmer for 8–10 minutes, until the carrots are just tender, basting occasionally. Taste, and add salt, if desired. 2. Transfer to a serving dish, spoon any juices on top, and sprinkle with parsley.

Per Serving

Calories: 48 | fat: 2.4g | protein: 0.66g | carbs: 6.49g | sugars: 2.76g | fiber: 2.3g | sodium: 46mg

Garlic Roasted Radishes

Prep time: 5 minutes | Cook time: 15 minutes | Serves 2 to 4

1 pound radishes, halved
1 tablespoon canola oil
Pinch kosher salt

4 garlic cloves, thinly sliced
¼ cup chopped fresh dill

1. Preheat the oven to 425°F. Line a baking sheet with parchment paper. 2. In a medium bowl, toss the radishes with the canola oil and salt. Spread the vegetables on the prepared baking sheet and roast for 10 minutes. Remove the sheet from the oven, add the garlic, mix well, and return to the oven for 5 minutes. 3. Remove the radishes from the oven, adjust the seasoning as desired, and serve topped with dill on a serving plate or as a side dish. 4. Store any leftovers in an airtight container in the refrigerator for 3 to 4 days.

Per Serving

Calories: 75 | fat: 4.85g | protein: 1.19g | carbs: 7.57g | sugars: 3.82g | fiber: 2.5g | sodium: 420mg

Ginger Broccoli

Prep time: 10 minutes | Cook time: 10 minutes | Serves 4

1 tablespoon extra-virgin olive oil
½ sweet onion, thinly sliced
2 teaspoons grated fresh ginger
1 teaspoon minced fresh garlic

2 heads broccoli, cut into small florets
¼ cup low-sodium chicken broth
Sea salt
Freshly ground black pepper

1. Place a large skillet over medium-high heat and add the oil. 2. Sauté the onion, ginger, and garlic until softened, about 3 minutes. 3. Add the broccoli florets and chicken broth, and sauté until the broccoli is tender, about 5 minutes. 4. Season with salt and pepper. 5. Serve immediately.

Per Serving

Calories: 240 | fat: 6g | protein: 17g | carbs: 41g | sugars: 12g | fiber: 15g | sodium: 341mg

Cheesy Cauli Bake

Prep time: 10 minutes | Cook time: 25 to 30 minutes | Serves 6

3 tablespoons tahini
2 tablespoons nutritional yeast
1 tablespoon lemon juice
½ teaspoon pure maple syrup or agave nectar
½ teaspoon sea salt
½ cup + 1 tablespoon plain nondairy milk

3–3½ cups cauliflower florets, cut or broken in small pieces
Topping
1 tablespoon almond meal or breadcrumbs
½ tablespoon nutritional yeast
Pinch sea salt

1. Preheat the oven to 425°F. Use cooking spray to lightly coat the bottom and sides of an 8" x 8" (or similar size) baking dish. 2. In a small bowl, whisk together the tahini, nutritional yeast, lemon juice, maple syrup or agave nectar, and salt. Gradually whisk in the milk until it all comes together smoothly. In the baking dish, add the cauliflower and pour in the sauce, stir thoroughly to coat the cauliflower. Cover with foil and bake for 25 to 30 minutes, stirring only once, until the cauliflower is tender. 3. In a small bowl, toss together the topping ingredients. Remove the foil from the cauliflower, and sprinkle on the topping. Return to the oven and set oven to broil. Allow to cook for a minute or so until the topping is golden brown. Remove, let sit for a few minutes, then serve.

Per Serving

Calorie: 87 | fat: 5g | protein: 5g | carbs: 7g | sugars: 5g | fiber: 3g | sodium: 270mg

Italian Wild Mushrooms

Prep time: 30 minutes | Cook time: 3 minutes | Serves 10

2 tablespoons canola oil
2 large onions, chopped
4 garlic cloves, minced
3 large red bell peppers, chopped
3 large green bell peppers, chopped
12-ounce package oyster

mushrooms, cleaned and chopped
3 fresh bay leaves
10 fresh basil leaves, chopped
1 teaspoon salt
1½ teaspoons pepper
28-ounce can Italian plum tomatoes, crushed or chopped

1. Press Sauté on the Instant Pot and add in the oil. Once the oil is heated, add the onions, garlic, peppers, and mushroom to the oil. Sauté just until mushrooms begin to turn brown. 2. Add remaining ingredients. Stir well. 3. Secure the lid and make sure vent is set to sealing. Press Manual and set time for 3 minutes. 4. When cook time is up, release the pressure manually. Discard bay leaves.

Per Serving

Calories: 82 | fat: 3g | protein: 3g | carbs: 13g | sugars: 8g | fiber: 4g | sodium: 356mg

Cauliflower and Butternut Squash Mac and Cheese

Prep time: 10 minutes | Cook time: 35 minutes | Serves 4

1 pound (454 g) chickpea pasta (any shape)
1 pound (454 g) cauliflower florets
1 (1-pounds [454-g]) butternut squash, peeled and cubed
1 teaspoon garlic powder

1 cup (240 ml) low-sodium vegetable broth
Sea salt, as needed
Black pepper, as needed
1 cup (120 g) shredded Cheddar cheese, divided

1. Preheat the oven to 400°F (204°C). 2. Bring two large pots of water to a boil over high heat. 3. Add the pasta to one pot of water and the cauliflower and butternut squash to the other. Cook the pasta according to the package directions and boil the vegetables for 10 to 12 minutes, until they are fork-tender. 4. Drain the pasta and transfer it to a large baking dish. 5. Drain the cauliflower and squash and transfer them to a high-power blender. Add the garlic powder, broth, sea salt, black pepper, and ¾ cup (90 g) of the Cheddar cheese. Blend until the sauce is smooth and creamy. 6. Pour the cheese sauce over the pasta and stir it to evenly distribute it throughout the pasta. Sprinkle the remaining ¼ cup (30 g) of Cheddar cheese over the top of the pasta. Bake the mac and cheese for 25 minutes, or until the cheese is melted and lightly browned.

Per Serving

Calorie: 388 | fat: 13g | protein: 25g | carbs: 43g | sugars: 10g | fiber: 13g | sodium: 315mg

Spicy Roasted Cauliflower with Lime

Prep time: 5 minutes | Cook time: 10 minutes | Serves 4

1 cauliflower head, broken into small florets
2 tablespoons extra-virgin olive oil

½ teaspoon ground chipotle chili powder
½ teaspoon salt
Juice of 1 lime

1. Preheat the oven to 450°F. Line a rimmed baking sheet with parchment paper. 2. In a large mixing bowl, toss the cauliflower with the olive oil, chipotle chili powder, and salt. Arrange in a single layer on the prepared baking sheet. 3. Roast for 15 minutes, flip, and continue to roast for 15 more minutes until well-browned and tender. 4. Sprinkle with the lime juice, adjust the salt as needed, and serve.

Per Serving

Calories: 99 | fat: 7 | protein: 3g | carbs: 8g | sugars: 3g | fiber: 3g | sodium: 284mg

Chapter 3 Staples, Sauces, Dips, and Dressings

Salsa Makeover   30

Thai-Style Peanut Sauce   30

Punchy Mustard Vinaigrette   30

Italian Turkey Sausage Meatballs   30

Vegetable broth   30

5-Minute Pesto   31

Roasted Red Pepper Spread   31

Green Chickpea Hummus   31

Ranch Vegetable Dip and Dressing   31

Not-So-Traditional Gravy   31

Ginger-Soy Dressing   32

Toasted Nuts   32

Ranch Dressing   32

Basic Marinara   32

Dreamy Caesar Dressing   32

Irresistible White Bean Dip   32

Orange Dijon Dressing   33

Low-Sodium Salsa   33

Salsa Makeover

Prep time: 5 minutes | Cook time: 0 minutes | Serves 5

1 cup store-bought fresh or jarred salsa
⅔ cup small cubes ripe avocado (about 1 avocado)
½ cup diced red pepper
½ cup frozen corn kernels, thawed in a bowl of boiled water

½ tablespoon lime juice
Few tablespoons chopped fresh cilantro or fresh parsley (optional)
Sea salt
Freshly ground pepper to taste (optional)

1. In a large bowl, combine the salsa, avocado, red pepper, corn, lime juice, and cilantro or parsley (if using). Mix together. Season to taste with salt and pepper, if using.

Per Serving

Calorie: 78 | fat: 4g | protein: 2g | carbs: 10g | sugars: 3g | fiber: 3g | sodium: 368mg

Thai-Style Peanut Sauce

Prep time: 10 minutes | Cook time: 0 minutes | Makes ⅔ cup

½ cup natural peanut butter
4 teaspoons sesame oil
2 tablespoons rice vinegar
1 teaspoon chopped peeled fresh ginger or pinch ground ginger
2 to 4 teaspoons freshly

squeezed lime juice, to your liking
2 to 2½ teaspoons hot sauce (optional)
1 teaspoon low-sodium soy sauce
1 teaspoon honey

1. In a small bowl, whisk together the peanut butter, sesame oil, and rice vinegar. The peanut butter will become more pliable as you whisk. 2. Whisk in the ginger. 3. Whisk in the lime juice, hot sauce (if using), soy sauce, and honey.

Per Serving⅓ cup:

Calorie: 473 | fat: 33g | protein: 19g | carbs: 30g | sugars: 10g | fiber: 4g | sodium: 471mg

Punchy Mustard Vinaigrette

Prep time: 5 minutes | Cook time: 0 minutes | Serves 6

¼ cup apple cider vinegar or rice vinegar
2 tablespoons tamari
1½ tablespoons yellow or Dijon mustard
2½ tablespoons coconut nectar

or pure maple syrup
½ tablespoon ground chia
Freshly ground black pepper to taste
⅛ teaspoon sea salt

1. In a blender, combine the vinegar, tamari, mustard, nectar or syrup, chia, pepper, and salt. Puree until fully incorporated. Taste, and add extra mustard if you love it! Season to taste with additional salt and pepper, if desired. Serve immediately or refrigerate. Dressing will keep for at least a week in the fridge.

Per Serving

Calorie: 33 | fat: 0g | protein: 1g | carbs: 7g | sugars: 5g | fiber: 1g | sodium: 428mg

Italian Turkey Sausage Meatballs

Prep time: 15 minutes | Cook time: 25 minutes | Makes About 24

1 pound ground chicken
8 ounces Italian turkey sausage (hot or sweet), casings removed
⅔ cup Italian-style breadcrumbs
2 teaspoons minced garlic
3 tablespoons chopped fresh

parsley
½ cup freshly grated Parmesan cheese
3 tablespoons nonfat milk
1 large egg, lightly beaten
1 teaspoon kosher salt
½ teaspoon freshly ground black pepper

1. Preheat the oven to 350ºF (180ºC). 2. In a large bowl, combine the chicken, sausage, bread crumbs, garlic, parsley, Parmesan, milk, egg, salt, and pepper. Mix gently but thoroughly. (I like to use my hands.) 3. Line a sheet pan with parchment paper. Pinch off about 1 tablespoon of the meat mixture and roll it into a ball. A 1¼-inch cookie scoop makes the job easy. Place the meatball on the sheet pan and repeat with the remaining meat. You should end up with about 24 meatballs. 4. If you plan to eat the meatballs right away, bake them for 30 minutes or until they are lightly browned and cooked through. If you plan to freeze the meatballs, bake them for 20 minutes, then let them cool before freezing.

Per Serving

Calorie: 64 | fat: 3g | protein: 6g | carbs: 3g | sugars: 1g | fiber: 0g | sodium: 254mg

Vegetable broth

Prep time: 10 minutes | Cook time: 15 minutes | Makes 8 Cups

2 or 3 (4-inch) rosemary sprigs
2 or 3 (4-inch) thyme sprigs
2 or 3 (4-inch) parsley sprigs
1 large onion (unpeeled), root end trimmed, quartered
2 large carrots (unpeeled), washed, ends trimmed, and each cut into 4 pieces

2 celery stalks (including leaves), ends trimmed and each cut into 4 pieces
4 garlic cloves, peeled and left whole
2 bay leaves
½ teaspoon peppercorns

1. Using kitchen twine, tie together the rosemary, thyme, and parsley. (If you don't have twine, don't worry about it. Tying the herbs together just makes it easier to discard them later.) 2. In the electric pressure cooker, combine the onion, carrots, celery, garlic, bay leaves, and peppercorns. Drop the herb bundle on top, then pour in 6 cups of water. 3. Close and lock the lid of the pressure cooker. Set the valve to sealing. 4. Cook on high pressure for 15 minutes. 5. When the cooking is complete, hit Cancel. Allow the pressure to release naturally for 15 minutes, then quick release any remaining pressure. 6. Once the pin drops, unlock and remove the lid. 7. Cool the broth to room temperature, then strain it through a fine-mesh strainer lined with cheesecloth. Discard the solids. 8. Transfer to storage containers and refrigerate for 3 to 4 days or freeze for up to 1 year.

Per Serving1 cup:

Calorie: 20 | fat: 0g | protein: 1g | carbs: 5g | sugars: 2g | fiber: 1g | sodium: 22mg

5-Minute Pesto

Prep time: 5 minutes | Cook time: 0 minutes | Makes 1 CUP

3 garlic cloves, peeled
2 cups packed fresh basil leaves
½ cup freshly grated Parmesan cheese

⅓ cup pine nuts
½ cup extra-virgin olive oil
Kosher salt
Freshly ground black pepper

1. With the motor running, drop the garlic cloves through the feed tube of a food processor fitted with the steel blade. Stop the motor, then add the basil, Parmesan, and pine nuts. Pulse a few times until the pine nuts are finely minced. 2. With the motor running, add the olive oil in a steady stream and process until the pesto is completely puréed. Season with salt and pepper.Store, covered, in the refrigerator for up to 2 weeks.

Per Serving⅛ cup:

Calorie: 175 | fat: 18g | protein: 2g | carbs: 1g | sugars: 0g | fiber: 0g | sodium: 96mg

Roasted Red Pepper Spread

Prep time: 5 minutes | Cook time: 0 minutes | Makes 1¼ cups

1 (16-ounce) jar roasted red bell peppers
1 cup canned low-sodium chickpeas, drained and rinsed
½ small jalapeño pepper, seeded and stemmed
2 tablespoons extra-virgin olive oil

2 tablespoons water
1 to 2 teaspoons freshly squeezed lime juice
½ teaspoon salt
¼ teaspoon garlic powder
¼ teaspoon ground cumin
⅛ teaspoon freshly ground black pepper

1. Put the bell peppers, chickpeas, jalapeño pepper, oil, water, lime juice, salt, garlic powder, cumin, and black pepper into a food processor or blender and blend until smooth. The sauce will have texture, but it shouldn't be chunky.

Per Serving¼ cup:

Calorie: 115 | fat: 7g | protein: 3g | carbs: 12g | sugars: 5g | fiber: 3g | sodium: 512mg

Green Chickpea Hummus

Prep time: 5 minutes | Cook time: 0 minutes | Serves 6

2 cups frozen green chickpeas
1 can (15 ounces) white beans, rinsed and drained
¼ cup lemon juice
1 large clove garlic (or more to taste)
⅓ cup fresh basil leaves
⅓ cup fresh parsley leaves

1 tablespoon tahini
1 teaspoon sea salt
½ teaspoon ground cumin
1–2 tablespoons water (optional)
½ teaspoon lemon zest (optional)

1. Add the chickpeas to a pot of boiling water and cook for just a minute to bring out their vibrant green color. Remove, run under cold water to stop the cooking process, and drain. In a food processor, combine the chickpeas, beans, lemon juice, garlic, basil, parsley, tahini, salt, and cumin. Puree until smooth, scraping down the bowl as needed. Add the water if desired to thin or help the pureeing process. Add the lemon zest, if desired, and season to taste. Serve.

Per Serving

Calorie: 176 | fat: 3g | protein: 10g | carbs: 29g | sugars: 3g | fiber: 8g | sodium: 477mg

Ranch Vegetable Dip and Dressing

Prep time: 10 minutes | Cook time: 0 minutes | Serves 8

2 cups frozen cauliflower, thawed
½ cup unsweetened plain almond milk
2 tablespoons extra-virgin olive oil
2 tablespoons apple cider vinegar
1 garlic clove, peeled
2 teaspoons finely chopped scallions, both white and green

parts
2 teaspoons finely chopped fresh parsley
1 teaspoon finely chopped fresh dill
½ teaspoon Dijon mustard
½ teaspoon onion powder
½ teaspoon salt
¼ teaspoon freshly ground black pepper

1. In a blender jar, combine the cauliflower, almond milk, oil, vinegar, garlic, scallions, parsley, dill, mustard, onion powder, salt, and pepper. Process until very smooth. 2. Serve immediately, or transfer to a jar, cover tightly with a lid, and store in the refrigerator for up to 3 days.

Per Serving

Calories: 42 | fat: 4g | protein: 1g | carbs: 2g | sugars: 1g | fiber: 1g | sodium: 149mg

Not-So-Traditional Gravy

Prep time: 5 minutes | Cook time: 15 minutes | Makes 1½ cups

2 cups store-bought low-sodium chicken broth, divided
4 tablespoons whole-wheat flour, divided
1 medium yellow onion, chopped
½ bunch fresh thyme, roughly

chopped
2 garlic cloves, minced
1 bay leaf
½ teaspoon celery seeds
Freshly ground black pepper
1 teaspoon Worcestershire sauce

1. In a shallow stockpot, combine ½ cup of broth and 1 tablespoon of whole-wheat flour and cook over medium-low heat, whisking until the flour is dissolved. Continue to add about ½ cup of broth and the remaining 3 tablespoons of flour in increments for about 2 minutes, or until a thick sauce is formed. 2. Add the onion, thyme, garlic, bay leaf, and ½ cup of broth, stirring well. 3. Add the celery seeds, pepper, Worcestershire sauce, and remaining ½ cup of broth. Stir and cook for 2 to 3 minutes, or until the gravy is thickened. Discard the bay leaf. 4. Serve spooned over your protein of choice.

Per Serving

Calorie: 86 | fat: 1g | protein: 5g | carbs: 15g | sugars: 2g | fiber: 3g | sodium: 70mg

Ginger-Soy Dressing

Prep time: 5 minutes | Cook time: 10 minutes | Serves 1

¼ cup light or reduced-sodium soy sauce
2 tablespoons sesame oil
2 tablespoons rice vinegar

1 tablespoon grated fresh ginger
1 tablespoon dry sherry
1 teaspoon light agave nectar

1. In a small jar, combine all ingredients. Cover the jar tightly, and shake vigorously until well blended. 2. Keep covered, and refrigerated until ready to serve. Shake again before serving.

Per Serving

Calorie: 81 | fat: 7g | protein: 1g | carbs: 3g | sugars: 2g | fiber: 0g | sodium: 576mg

Toasted Nuts

Prep time: 1 minutes | Cook time: 8 minutes | Makes ½ CUP

½ cup nuts

1. Heat a dry nonstick pan over medium-high heat. 2. Place the nuts in the pan and toss or stir frequently for 2 to 5 minutes, until they are toasted and fragrant. 3. Remove from the heat and let cool.

Per Serving

Calorie: 346 | fat: 27g | protein: 13g | carbs: 17g | sugars: 5g | fiber: 7g | sodium: 1mg

Ranch Dressing

Prep time: 10 minutes | Cook time: 0 minutes | Serves 8 to 10

8 ounces fat-free plain Greek yogurt
¼ cup low-fat buttermilk
1 tablespoon garlic powder
1 tablespoon dried dill

1 tablespoon dried chives
1 tablespoon onion powder
1 tablespoon dried parsley
Pinch freshly ground black pepper

1. In a shallow, medium bowl, combine the Greek yogurt and buttermilk. 2. Stir in the garlic powder, dill, chives, onion powder, parsley, and pepper and mix well. 3. Serve with animal protein or vegetable of your choice, or place in an airtight container.

Per Serving

Calorie: 24 | fat: 0g | protein: 3g | carbs: 3g | sugars: 1g | fiber: 0g | sodium: 21mg

Basic Marinara

Prep time: 5 minutes | Cook time: 25 minutes | Makes 8 cups

¼ cup extra-virgin olive oil
1 small onion, minced
4 garlic cloves, thinly sliced
2 basil sprigs
1 teaspoon dried oregano

2 (28-ounce) cans diced or crushed tomatoes
Kosher salt
Freshly ground pepper

1. Heat the extra-virgin olive oil in a medium heavy stockpot over medium heat. Cook the onion, stirring occasionally, until very soft, 3 to 5 minutes. 2. Add the garlic and cook, stirring occasionally, until very soft, about 5 minutes. Add the basil and oregano and stir to combine. 3. Add the tomatoes and bring to a simmer. Reduce the heat to low and simmer, stirring occasionally, until the sauce is thick, about 15 minutes. 4. Season with salt and pepper. 5. Store in an airtight container in the refrigerator for up to 1 week or in the freezer for up to 3 months.

Per Serving1 cup:

Calorie: 99 | fat: 7g | protein: 2g | carbs: 9g | sugars: 6g | fiber: 4g | sodium: 22mg

Dreamy Caesar Dressing

Prep time: 10 minutes | Cook time: 0 minutes | Serves 12

¼–⅓ cup soaked almonds or cashews
½ cup cooked red or yellow potato, skins removed
2 tablespoons freshly squeezed lemon juice
1½ tablespoons red wine vinegar
1 medium or large clove garlic, chopped (adjust to taste)
1 tablespoon chickpea miso (or

other mild-flavored miso)
2 teaspoons Dijon mustard
½ teaspoon sea salt
Freshly ground black pepper to taste
1 teaspoon pure maple syrup
¾ cup plain low-fat nondairy milk
2–3 tablespoons water or nondairy milk (optional)

1. In a blender, combine the nuts, potato, lemon juice, vinegar, garlic, miso, mustard, salt, pepper, syrup, and milk. Puree until very smooth. Add the water or additional milk to thin the dressing, if desired. (It will thicken after refrigeration.)

Per Serving

Calorie: 34 | fat: 2g | protein: 1g | carbs: 4g | sugars: 1g | fiber: 1g | sodium: 177mg

Irresistible White Bean Dip

Prep time: 5 minutes | Cook time: 0 minutes | Serves 4

1 can (15 ounces) white beans, rinsed and drained
2 tablespoons lemon juice
2 teaspoons miso
Scant ½ teaspoon sea salt
¼ teaspoon black salt

1 tablespoon tahini
1 tablespoon nutritional yeast
1 clove garlic (or to taste)
¼–½ teaspoon pure maple syrup (optional)
1–1½ tablespoons water

1. In a small food processor or high-powered blender, combine the beans, lemon juice, miso, sea salt, black salt, tahini, yeast, garlic, syrup (if using), and 1 tablespoon of the water. Puree, adding the additional ½ tablespoon water if needed. (Just don't add too much; the dip should be thick.) Taste, and season with extra lemon, salt, or garlic, if desired.

Per Serving

Calorie: 139 | fat: 3g | protein: 9g | carbs: 21g | sugars: 1g | fiber: 6g | sodium: 638mg

Orange Dijon Dressing

Prep time: 5 minutes | Cook time: 0 minutes | Serves 2

¼ cup extra-virgin olive oil
2 tablespoons freshly squeezed orange juice
1 orange, zested
1 teaspoon garlic powder

¾ teaspoon za'atar seasoning
½ teaspoon salt
¼ teaspoon Dijon mustard
Freshly ground black pepper, to taste

1. In a jar, combine the olive oil, orange juice and zest, garlic powder, za'atar, salt, and mustard. Season with pepper and shake vigorously until completely mixed.

Per Serving

Calorie: 284 | fat: 27g | protein: 1g | carbs: 11g | sugars: 8g | fiber: 2g | sodium: 590mg

Low-Sodium Salsa

Prep time: 10 minutes | Cook time: 10 minutes | Makes 1 CUP

8 ounces cocktail tomatoes, quartered
2 scallions, white and light green parts only, chopped
1 jalapeño chile, seeded and chopped

2 tablespoons chopped fresh cilantro
1 tablespoon freshly squeezed lime juice

1. In a food processor, combine the tomatoes, scallions, jalapeño, cilantro, and lime juice. Pulse until the salsa is the consistency you like. If you don't have a food processor, finely chop the tomatoes, scallions, and jalapeño, then mix with the cilantro and lime juice. 2. Store, covered, in the refrigerator for up to 3 days.

Per Serving¼ cup:

Calorie: 12 | fat: 0g | protein: 1g | carbs: 3g | sugars: 2g | fiber: 1g | sodium: 3mg

Chapter 4 Beef, Pork, and Lamb

Smothered Sirloin   35

Beef Burgundy   35

Italian Sausages with Peppers and
Onions   35

Asian Steak Salad   35

Salisbury Steaks with Seared
Cauliflower   36

Slow Cooker Ropa Vieja   36

Grilled Steak and Vegetables   36

Pork Mole Quesadillas   37

Mediterranean Steak Sandwiches   37

Zesty Swiss Steak   37

Herbed Chipotle Pot Roast   37

Mustard Herb Pork Tenderloin   38

Homey Pot Roast   38

Quick Steak Tacos   38

Garlic Beef Stroganoff   38

Tenderloin with Crispy Shallots   39

Steak with Bell Pepper   39

Traditional Beef Stroganoff   39

Mango-Glazed Pork Tenderloin
Roast   39

Dutch Oven Apple Pork Chops   40

Open-Faced Pulled Pork   40

Steak Gyro Platter   40

Short Ribs with Chimichurri   40

Red Wine Pot Roast with Winter
Vegetables   41

Sage-Parmesan Pork Chops   41

Spiced Lamb Stew   41

Creole Steak   42

Slow-Cooked Simple Lamb and
Vegetable Stew   42

Italian Beef Kebabs   42

Spinach and Provolone Steak Rolls   42

Roasted Beef with Peppercorn
Sauce   43

Slow-Cooked Pork Burrito Bowls   43

Herb-Crusted Lamb Chops   43

Easy Pot Roast and Vegetables   43

Steak Fajita Bake   44

Beef and Vegetable Shish Kabobs   44

Lamb Kofta Meatballs with Cucumber
Quick-Pickled Salad   44

Lamb Chops with Cherry Glaze   44

Sloppy Joes   44

Pork Butt Roast   45

Beef Stew   45

Rosemary Roast Beef   45

Pork Tenderloin Stir-Fry   45

Mediterranean Beef Steaks   46

Butterflied Beef Eye Roast   46

Smothered Sirloin

Prep time: 15 minutes | Cook time: 30 minutes | Serves 5

1 pound beef round sirloin tip
1 teaspoon freshly ground black pepper
1 teaspoon celery seeds
2 tablespoons extra-virgin olive oil
1 medium yellow onion, chopped
¼ cup chickpea flour
2 cups store-bought low-sodium chicken broth, divided
2 celery stalks, thinly sliced

1 medium red bell pepper, chopped
2 garlic cloves, minced
2 tablespoons whole-wheat flour
Generous pinch cayenne pepper
Chopped fresh chives, for garnish (optional)
Smoked paprika, for garnish (optional)

1. In a bowl, season the steak on both sides with the black pepper and celery seeds. 2. Select the Sauté setting on an electric pressure cooker, and combine the olive oil and onions. Cook for 3 to 5 minutes, stirring, or until the onions are browned but not burned. 3. Slowly add the chickpea flour, 1 tablespoon at a time, while stirring. 4. Add 1 cup of broth, ¼ cup at a time, as needed. 5. Stir in the celery, bell pepper, and garlic and cook for 3 to 5 minutes, or until softened. 6. Lay the beef on top of vegetables, and pour the remaining 1 cup of broth on top. 7. Close and lock the lid and set the pressure valve to sealing. 8. Change to the Manual/Pressure Cook setting, and cook for 20 minutes. 9. Once cooking is complete, quick-release the pressure. Carefully remove the lid. 10. Remove the steak and vegetables from the pressure cooker, reserving the leftover liquid for the gravy base. 11. To make the gravy, add the whole-wheat flour and cayenne to the liquid in the pressure cooker, mixing continuously until thickened. 12. To serve, spoon the gravy over the steak and garnish with the chives (if using) and paprika (if using).

Per Serving

Calorie: 234 | fat: 11g | protein: 23g | carbs: 11g | sugars: 3g | fiber: 2g | sodium: 96mg

Beef Burgundy

Prep time: 30 minutes | Cook time: 30 minutes | Serves 6

2 tablespoons olive oil
2 pounds stewing meat, cubed, trimmed of fat
2½ tablespoons flour
5 medium onions, thinly sliced
½ pound fresh mushrooms, sliced

1 teaspoon salt
¼ teaspoon dried marjoram
¼ teaspoon dried thyme
⅛ teaspoon pepper
¾ cup beef broth
1½ cups burgundy

1. Press Sauté on the Instant pot and add in the olive oil. 2. Dredge meat in flour, then brown in batches in the Instant Pot. Set aside the meat. Sauté the onions and mushrooms in the remaining oil and drippings for about 3–4 minutes, then add the meat back in. Press Cancel. 3. Add the salt, marjoram, thyme, pepper, broth, and wine to the Instant Pot. 4. Secure the lid and make sure the vent is set to sealing. Press the Manual button and set to 30 minutes. 5. When cook time is up, let the pressure release naturally for 15 minutes, then perform a quick release. 6.

Serve over cooked noodles.

Per Serving

Calories: 358 | fat: 11g | protein: 37g | carbs: 15g | sugars: 5g | fiber: 2g | sodium: 472mg

Italian Sausages with Peppers and Onions

Prep time: 5 minutes | Cook time: 28 minutes | Serves 3

1 medium onion, thinly sliced
1 yellow or orange bell pepper, thinly sliced
1 red bell pepper, thinly sliced
¼ cup avocado oil or melted

coconut oil
1 teaspoon fine sea salt
6 Italian sausages
Dijon mustard, for serving (optional)

1. Preheat the air fryer to 400°F (204°C). 2. Place the onion and peppers in a large bowl. Drizzle with the oil and toss well to coat the veggies. Season with the salt. 3. Place the onion and peppers in a pie pan and cook in the air fryer for 8 minutes, stirring halfway through. Remove from the air fryer and set aside. 4. Spray the air fryer basket with avocado oil. Place the sausages in the air fryer basket and air fry for 20 minutes, or until crispy and golden brown. During the last minute or two of cooking, add the onion and peppers to the basket with the sausages to warm them through. 5. Place the onion and peppers on a serving platter and arrange the sausages on top. Serve Dijon mustard on the side, if desired. 6. Store leftovers in an airtight container in the fridge for up to 7 days or in the freezer for up to a month. Reheat in a preheated 390°F (199°C) air fryer for 3 minutes, or until heated through.

Per Serving

Calorie: 455 | fat: 33g | protein: 29g | carbs: 13g | sugars: 3g | fiber: 2g | sodium: 392mg

Asian Steak Salad

Prep time: 20 minutes | Cook time: 5 minutes | Serves 6

1 pound cut-up lean beef for stir-fry
1 package (3 ounces) Oriental-flavor ramen noodle soup mix
½ cup low-fat Asian marinade and dressing
1 bag (10 ounces) romaine and

leaf lettuce mix
1 cup fresh snow pea pods
½ cup matchstick-cut carrots (from 10-ounce bag)
1 can (11 ounces) mandarin orange segments, drained

1. Spray 12-inch skillet with cooking spray; heat over medium-high heat. Place beef in skillet; sprinkle with 1 teaspoon seasoning mix from soup mix. (Discard remaining seasoning mix.) Cook beef 4 to 5 minutes, stirring occasionally, until brown. Stir in 1 tablespoon of the dressing. 2. Break block of noodles from soup mix into small pieces. Mix noodles, lettuce, pea pods, carrots, and orange segments in large bowl. Add remaining dressing; toss until well coated. Divide mixture among 6 serving plates. Top with beef.

Per Serving

Calories: 240 | fat: 7g | protein: 19g | carbs: 25g | sugars: 14g | fiber: 2g | sodium: 990mg

Salisbury Steaks with Seared Cauliflower

Prep time: 5 minutes | Cook time: 30 minutes | Serves 4

Salisbury Steaks
1 pound 95 percent lean ground beef
⅓ cup almond flour
1 large egg
½ teaspoon fine sea salt
¼ teaspoon freshly ground black pepper
2 tablespoons cold-pressed avocado oil
1 small yellow onion, sliced
1 garlic clove, chopped
8 ounces cremini or button mushrooms, sliced

½ teaspoon fine sea salt
2 tablespoons tomato paste
1½ teaspoons yellow mustard
1 cup low-sodium roasted beef bone broth
Seared Cauliflower
1 tablespoon olive oil
1 head cauliflower, cut into bite-size florets
2 tablespoons chopped fresh flat-leaf parsley
¼ teaspoon fine sea salt
2 teaspoons cornstarch
2 teaspoons water

1. To make the steaks: In a bowl, combine the beef, almond flour, egg, salt, and pepper and mix with your hands until all of the ingredients are evenly distributed. Divide the mixture into four equal portions, then shape each portion into an oval patty about ½ inch thick. 2. Select the Sauté setting on the Instant Pot and heat the oil for 2 minutes. Swirl the oil to coat the bottom of the pot, then add the patties and sear for 3 minutes, until browned on one side. Using a thin, flexible spatula, flip the patties and sear the second side for 2 to 3 minutes, until browned. Transfer the patties to a plate. 3. Add the onion, garlic, mushrooms, and salt to the pot and sauté for 4 minutes, until the onion is translucent and the mushrooms have begun to give up their liquid. Add the tomato paste, mustard, and broth and stir with a wooden spoon, using it to nudge any browned bits from the bottom of the pot. Return the patties to the pot in a single layer and spoon a bit of the sauce over each one. 4. Secure the lid and set the Pressure Release to Sealing. Press the Cancel button to reset the cooking program, then select the Pressure Cook or Manual setting and set the cooking time for 10 minutes at high pressure. (The pot will take about 5 minutes to come up to pressure before the cooking program begins.) 5. When the cooking program ends, let the pressure release naturally for at least 10 minutes, then move the Pressure Release to Venting to release any remaining steam. 6. To make the cauliflower: While the pressure is releasing, in a large skillet over medium heat, warm the oil. Add the cauliflower and stir or toss to coat with the oil, then cook, stirring every minute or two, until lightly browned, about 8 minutes. Turn off the heat, sprinkle in the parsley and salt, and stir to combine. Leave in the skillet, uncovered, to keep warm. 7. Open the pot and, using a slotted spatula, transfer the patties to a serving plate. In a small bowl, stir together the cornstarch and water. Press the Cancel button to reset the cooking program, then select the Sauté setting. When the sauce comes to a simmer, stir in the cornstarch mixture and let the sauce boil for about 1 minute, until thickened. Press the Cancel button to turn off the Instant Pot. 8. Spoon the sauce over the patties. Serve right away, with the cauliflower.

Per Serving

Calorie: 362 | fat: 21g | protein: 33g | carbs: 21g | sugars: 4g | fiber: 6g | sodium: 846mg

Slow Cooker Ropa Vieja

Prep time: 5 minutes | Cook time: 20 minutes | Serves 4

½ small yellow onion
1 red bell pepper
1 (14-ounce) can no-salt-added diced tomatoes
1 teaspoon dried oregano
½ teaspoon salt

½ teaspoon smoked paprika
½ teaspoon garlic powder
1 pound chuck beef roast, trimmed of visible fat
1 head cauliflower

1. Cut the onion and bell pepper into ½-inch-thick slices. 2. Place the onion, bell pepper, diced tomatoes with their juices, oregano, salt, paprika, and garlic powder in a slow cooker, then add the beef. 3. Place the head of cauliflower on top of the beef, and cook on low for 8 hours. 4. When fully cooked, the cauliflower will fall apart when scooped.

Per Serving

Calorie: 22- | fat: 7g | protein: 27g | carbs: 14g | sugars: 7g | fiber: 6g | sodium: 445mg

Grilled Steak and Vegetables

Prep time: 15 minutes | Cook time: 25 minutes | Serves 2

Extra-virgin olive oil cooking spray
2 (8-ounce) sirloin steaks
2 medium pear-shaped tomatoes, halved lengthwise
1 medium zucchini, cut into chunks
1 medium yellow squash, cut into chunks
1 bell pepper (any color), cut

into 1-inch pieces
2 tablespoons extra-virgin olive oil, divided
1 garlic clove, minced
¼ cup fresh basil, plus fresh sprigs, for garnish
Pinch salt
Freshly ground black pepper, to season

1. Preheat the grill (charcoal or gas). 2. Lightly coat a grill rack with cooking spray. 3. Place the steaks on the grill rack, about 4 to 6 inches above the heat—whether a solid bed of medium-hot coals or gas. Cook for about 15 minutes, turning as needed, until evenly browned on the outside and an instant-read thermometer inserted in the center registers 145°F for medium-rare. 4. While the steaks cook, place the tomatoes, zucchini, yellow squash, and bell pepper on the grill. Brush lightly with 1 tablespoon of olive oil. Grill for about 3 minutes, or until the vegetables are browned on the bottom. Turn them over. Continue to cook for about 3 minutes more, or until soft. 5. In a medium skillet with a heatproof handle set over medium-high heat, stir together the remaining 1 tablespoon of olive oil, garlic, and basil. 6. Transfer the grilled vegetables to the skillet. Stir to combine. Reduce the heat to low. 7. Serve each steak accompanied by half of the vegetables. Season with salt and pepper. Garnish with the basil sprigs.

Per Serving

Calorie: 631 | fat: 38g | protein: 52g | carbs: 18g | sugars: 8g | fiber: 5g | sodium: 239mg

Pork Mole Quesadillas

Prep time: 35 minutes | Cook time: 15 minutes | Makes 4 quesadillas

2 teaspoons canola oil
½ pound boneless pork loin chops, trimmed of fat, cut into thin strips
1 medium green bell pepper, thinly sliced
1 medium red bell pepper, thinly sliced
1 medium onion, thinly sliced
3 cloves garlic, finely chopped
1 tablespoon chili powder
1 teaspoon all-purpose flour
1 teaspoon ground cumin
¼ teaspoon salt
¼ teaspoon ground cinnamon
¼ cup reduced-sodium chicken broth
2 tablespoons semisweet chocolate chips
4 fat-free flour tortillas (10 inch)
Cooking spray
½ cup chopped tomato
4 teaspoons chopped fresh cilantro
½ cup shredded reduced-fat Monterey Jack cheese (2 ounces)

1. In 12-inch nonstick skillet, heat 1 teaspoon of the oil over medium-high heat. Add pork to oil. Cook 4 to 5 minutes, stirring frequently, until pork is no longer pink; remove from skillet. 2. In same skillet, heat remaining 1 teaspoon oil over medium heat. Add bell peppers, onion and garlic to oil. Cook 3 to 5 minutes, stirring occasionally, until bell peppers are crisp-tender. Stir in chili powder, flour, cumin, salt and cinnamon; cook 30 seconds. Stir in chicken broth; heat to boiling. Cook about 30 seconds, stirring constantly, until thickened and bubbly. Remove from heat; stir in chocolate chips until melted. Stir in pork. 3. Spray 1 side of each tortilla with cooking spray. On work surface, place tortillas, sprayed side down. Arrange pork mixture, tomato, cilantro and cheese evenly over half of each tortilla. Fold tortilla over filling, pressing gently. 4. Heat 12-inch skillet over medium heat until hot. Cook 2 quesadillas 3 to 4 minutes, turning once, until tortillas begin to brown; remove quesadillas from pan. Keep warm. Repeat with remaining 2 quesadillas. 5. To serve, cut into wedges, beginning from center of folded side.

Per Serving1 Quesadilla:

Calories: 450 | fat: 17g | protein: 23g | carbs: 40g | sugars: 8g | fiber: 4g | sodium: 810mg

Mediterranean Steak Sandwiches

Prep time: 10 minutes | Cook time: 10 minutes | Serves 4

2 tablespoons extra-virgin olive oil
2 tablespoons balsamic vinegar
2 teaspoons minced garlic
2 teaspoons freshly squeezed lemon juice
2 teaspoons chopped fresh oregano
1 teaspoon chopped fresh parsley
1 pound flank steak, trimmed of fat
4 whole-wheat pitas
2 cups shredded lettuce
1 red onion, thinly sliced
1 tomato, chopped
1 ounce low-sodium feta cheese

1. In a large bowl, whisk together the olive oil, balsamic vinegar, garlic, lemon juice, oregano, and parsley. 2. Add the steak to the bowl, turning to coat it completely. 3. Marinate the steak for 1 hour in the refrigerator, turning it over several times. 4. Preheat the broiler. Line a baking sheet with aluminum foil. 5. Take the steak out of the bowl and discard the marinade. 6. Place the steak on the baking sheet and broil until it is done to your liking, about 5 minutes per side for medium. 7. Let the steak rest for 10 minutes before slicing it thinly on a bias. 8. Stuff the pitas with the sliced steak, lettuce, onion, tomato, and feta.

Per Serving

Calorie: 331 | fat: 15g | protein: 30g | carbs: 20g | sugars: 3g | fiber: 3g | sodium: 191mg

Zesty Swiss Steak

Prep time: 35 minutes | Cook time: 35 minutes | Serves 6

3–4 tablespoons flour
½ teaspoon salt
¼ teaspoon pepper
1½ teaspoons dry mustard
1½–2 pounds round steak, trimmed of fat
1 tablespoon canola oil
1 cup sliced onions
1 pound carrots, sliced
14½-ounce can whole tomatoes
⅓ cup water
1 tablespoon brown sugar
1½ tablespoons Worcestershire sauce

1. Combine flour, salt, pepper, and dry mustard. 2. Cut steak in serving pieces. Dredge in flour mixture. 3. Set the Instant Pot to Sauté and add in the oil. Brown the steak pieces on both sides in the oil. Press Cancel. 4. Add onions and carrots into the Instant Pot. 5. Combine the tomatoes, water, brown sugar, and Worcestershire sauce. Pour into the Instant Pot. 6. Secure the lid and make sure the vent is set to sealing. Press Manual and set the time for 35 minutes. 7. When cook time is up, let the pressure release naturally for 15 minutes, then perform a quick release.

Per Serving

Calories: 236 | fat: 8g | protein: 23g | carbs: 18g | sugars: 9g | fiber: 3g | sodium: 426mg

Herbed Chipotle Pot Roast

Prep time: 5 minutes | Cook time: 3 hours | Serves 5

1 tablespoon extra-virgin olive oil
One 2-pound lean boneless beef roast
⅛ teaspoon freshly ground black pepper
½ cup water
⅓ cup dry sherry
¼ cup chipotle sauce
1 garlic clove, minced
¼ teaspoon dried rosemary
¼ teaspoon dried thyme
2 medium onions, sliced
1 bay leaf
1 cup sliced mushrooms

1. Add the olive oil to a large Dutch oven over medium heat. Sprinkle the roast with the pepper; brown the roast on all sides. 2. Combine the water, sherry, chipotle, garlic, rosemary, and thyme in a small bowl, and pour over the roast. Add the onions and bay leaf, cover, and simmer for 2–3 hours, until the roast is tender. 3. During the last 15 minutes, add the mushrooms, and continue simmering until heated. Remove the bay leaf. Transfer the roast to a platter, slice, and serve.

Per Serving

Calorie: 288 | fat: 13g | protein: 38g | carbs: 5g | sugars: 2g | fiber: 1g | sodium: 233mg

Mustard Herb Pork Tenderloin

Prep time: 5 minutes | Cook time: 20 minutes | Serves 6

¼ cup mayonnaise
2 tablespoons Dijon mustard
½ teaspoon dried thyme
¼ teaspoon dried rosemary
1 (1-pound / 454-g) pork

tenderloin
½ teaspoon salt
¼ teaspoon ground black
pepper

1. In a small bowl, mix mayonnaise, mustard, thyme, and rosemary. Brush tenderloin with mixture on all sides, then sprinkle with salt and pepper on all sides. 2. Place tenderloin into ungreased air fryer basket. Adjust the temperature to 400°F (204°C) and air fry for 20 minutes, turning tenderloin halfway through cooking. Tenderloin will be golden and have an internal temperature of at least 145°F (63°C) when done. Serve warm.

Per Serving

Calorie: 118 | fat: 5g | protein: 17g | carbs: 1g | sugars: 0g | fiber: 0g | sodium: 368mg

Homey Pot Roast

Prep time: 15 minutes | Cook time: 2 hour 15 minutes | Serves 6

1 pound boneless beef chuck
roast
2 tablespoons Creole
seasoning
2 cups store-bought low-
sodium chicken broth, divided
1 large portobello mushroom,
cut into 2-inch pieces
1 small onion, roughly
chopped
3 celery stalks, roughly
chopped
4 medium tomatoes, chopped

2 garlic cloves, minced
1 medium green pepper,
roughly chopped
8 ounces steamer potatoes,
skin on, halved
6 small parsnips, peeled and
halved
2 large carrots, peeled and cut
into 2-inch pieces
3 bay leaves
Freshly ground black pepper
Pinch cayenne pepper
Pinch smoked paprika

1. Preheat the oven to 325°F. 2. Massage the roast all over with the Creole seasoning. 3. In a Dutch oven, bring ½ cup of broth to a simmer over medium heat. 4. Add the beef and cook on all sides, turning to avoid burning the meat, no more than about 2½ minutes per side, or until browned. Remove the beef from the pot and set aside. 5. Add the mushroom, onion, celery, tomatoes, garlic, and green pepper to pot, adding up to ½ cup of broth if needed to prevent blackening of the vegetables. 6. Reduce the heat to medium-low and cook, stirring continuously, for 5 to 7 minutes, or until the vegetables have softened. 7. Return the beef to the pot. Add the potatoes, parsnips, carrots, bay leaves, and remaining 1 cup of broth. 8. Season with the black pepper, cayenne, and paprika. 9. Cover the pot, transfer to the oven, and bake for 2 hours, or until the beef is juicy and falls apart easily. Discard the bay leaves. 10. Serve.

Per Serving

Calorie: 237 | fat: 5g | protein: 20g | carbs: 29g | sugars: 8g | fiber: 7g | sodium: 329mg

Quick Steak Tacos

Prep time: 5 minutes | Cook time: 10 minutes | Serves 6

1 tablespoon olive oil
8 ounces sirloin steak
2 tablespoons steak seasoning
1 teaspoon Worcestershire
sauce
½ red onion, halved and sliced
6 corn tortillas
¼ cup tomatoes

¾ cup reduced-fat Mexican
cheese
2 tablespoons low-fat sour
cream
6 tablespoons garden fresh
salsa
¼ cup chopped fresh cilantro

1. Turn the Instant Pot on the Sauté function. When the pot displays "hot," add the olive oil to the pot. 2. Season the steak with the steak seasoning. 3. Add the steak to the pot along with the Worcestershire sauce. 4. Cook each side of the steak for 2–3 minutes until the steak turns brown. 5. Remove the steak from the pot and slice thinly. 6. Add the onion to the pot with the remaining olive oil and steak juices and cook them until translucent. 7. Remove the onion from the pot. 8. Warm your corn tortillas, then assemble your steak, onion, tomatoes, cheese, sour cream, salsa, and cilantro on top of each.

Per Serving

Calories: 187 | fat: 9g | protein: 14g | carbs: 14g | sugars: 2g | fiber: 2g | sodium: 254mg

Garlic Beef Stroganoff

Prep time: 20 minutes | Cook time: 25 minutes | Serves 6

2 tablespoons canola oil
1½ pounds boneless round
steak, cut into thin strips,
trimmed of fat
2 teaspoons sodium-free beef
bouillon powder
1 cup mushroom juice, with
water added to make a full cup
2 (4½-ounce) jars sliced
mushrooms, drained with juice

reserved
10¾-ounce can 98% fat-
free, lower-sodium cream of
mushroom soup
1 large onion, chopped
3 garlic cloves, minced
1 tablespoon Worcestershire
sauce
6-ounces fat-free cream
cheese, cubed and softened

1. Press the Sauté button and put the oil into the Instant Pot inner pot. 2. Once the oil is heated, sauté the beef until it is lightly browned, about 2 minutes on each side. Set the beef aside for a moment. Press Cancel and wipe out the Instant Pot with some paper towel. 3. Press Sauté again and dissolve the bouillon in the mushroom juice and water in inner pot of the Instant Pot. Once dissolved, press Cancel. 4. Add the mushrooms, soup, onion, garlic, and Worcestershire sauce and stir. Add the beef back to the pot. 5. Secure the lid and make sure the vent is set to sealing. Press Manual and set for 15 minutes. 6. When cook time is up, let the pressure release naturally for 15 minutes, then perform a quick release. 7. Press Cancel and remove the lid. Press Sauté. Stir in cream cheese until smooth. 8. Serve over noodles.

Per Serving

Calories: 202 | fat: 8g | protein: 21g | carbs: 10g | sugars: 4g | fiber: 2g | sodium: 474mg

Tenderloin with Crispy Shallots

Prep time: 30 minutes | Cook time: 18 to 20 minutes | Serves 6

1½ pounds (680 g) beef tenderloin steaks
Sea salt and freshly ground black pepper, to taste
4 medium shallots
1 teaspoon olive oil or avocado oil

1. Season both sides of the steaks with salt and pepper, and let them sit at room temperature for 45 minutes. 2. Set the air fryer to 400ºF (204ºC) and let it preheat for 5 minutes. 3. Working in batches if necessary, place the steaks in the air fryer basket in a single layer and air fry for 5 minutes. Flip and cook for 5 minutes longer, until an instant-read thermometer inserted in the center of the steaks registers 120ºF (49ºC) for medium-rare (or as desired). Remove the steaks and tent with aluminum foil to rest. 4. Set the air fryer to 300ºF (149ºC). In a medium bowl, toss the shallots with the oil. Place the shallots in the basket and air fry for 5 minutes, then give them a toss and cook for 3 to 5 minutes more, until crispy and golden brown. 5. Place the steaks on serving plates and arrange the shallots on top.

Per Serving

Calorie: 166 | fat: 8g | protein: 24g | carbs: 1g | sugars: 0g | fiber: 0g | sodium: 72mg

Steak with Bell Pepper

Prep time: 30 minutes | Cook time: 20 to 23 minutes | Serves 6

¼ cup avocado oil
¼ cup freshly squeezed lime juice
2 teaspoons minced garlic
1 tablespoon chili powder
½ teaspoon ground cumin
Sea salt and freshly ground black pepper, to taste
1 pound (454 g) top sirloin
steak or flank steak, thinly sliced against the grain
1 red bell pepper, cored, seeded, and cut into ½-inch slices
1 green bell pepper, cored, seeded, and cut into ½-inch slices
1 large onion, sliced

1. In a small bowl or blender, combine the avocado oil, lime juice, garlic, chili powder, cumin, and salt and pepper to taste. 2. Place the sliced steak in a zip-top bag or shallow dish. Place the bell peppers and onion in a separate zip-top bag or dish. Pour half the marinade over the steak and the other half over the vegetables. Seal both bags and let the steak and vegetables marinate in the refrigerator for at least 1 hour or up to 4 hours. 3. Line the air fryer basket with an air fryer liner or aluminum foil. Remove the vegetables from their bag or dish and shake off any excess marinade. Set the air fryer to 400ºF (204ºC). Place the vegetables in the air fryer basket and cook for 13 minutes. 4. Remove the steak from its bag or dish and shake off any excess marinade. Place the steak on top of the vegetables in the air fryer, and cook for 7 to 10 minutes or until an instant-read thermometer reads 120ºF (49ºC) for medium-rare (or cook to your desired doneness). 5. Serve with desired fixings, such as keto tortillas, lettuce, sour cream, avocado slices, shredded Cheddar cheese, and cilantro.

Per Serving

Calorie: 252 | fat: 18g | protein: 17g | carbs: 6g | sugars: 3g | fiber: 2g | sodium: 81mg

Traditional Beef Stroganoff

Prep time: 10 minutes | Cook time: 30 minutes | Serves 4

1 teaspoon extra-virgin olive oil
1 pound top sirloin, cut into thin strips
1 cup sliced button mushrooms
½ sweet onion, finely chopped
1 teaspoon minced garlic
1 tablespoon whole-wheat
flour
½ cup low-sodium beef broth
¼ cup dry sherry
½ cup fat-free sour cream
1 tablespoon chopped fresh parsley
Sea salt
Freshly ground black pepper

1. Place a large skillet over medium-high heat and add the oil. 2. Sauté the beef until browned, about 10 minutes, then remove the beef with a slotted spoon to a plate and set it aside. 3. Add the mushrooms, onion, and garlic to the skillet and sauté until lightly browned, about 5 minutes. 4. Whisk in the flour and then whisk in the beef broth and sherry. 5. Return the sirloin to the skillet and bring the mixture to a boil. 6. Reduce the heat to low and simmer until the beef is tender, about 10 minutes. 7. Stir in the sour cream and parsley. Season with salt and pepper.

Per Serving

Calorie: 320 | fat: 18g | protein: 26g | carbs: 13g | sugars: 3g | fiber: 1g | sodium: 111mg

Mango-Glazed Pork Tenderloin Roast

Prep time: 10 minutes | Cook time: 20 minutes | Serves 4

1 pound boneless pork tenderloin, trimmed of fat
1 teaspoon chopped fresh rosemary
1 teaspoon chopped fresh thyme
¼ teaspoon salt, divided
¼ teaspoon freshly ground black pepper, divided
1 teaspoon extra-virgin olive
oil
1 tablespoon honey
2 tablespoons white wine vinegar
2 tablespoons dry cooking wine
1 tablespoon minced fresh ginger
1 cup diced mango

1. Preheat the oven to 400°F. 2. Season the tenderloin with the rosemary, thyme, ⅛ teaspoon of salt, and ⅛ teaspoon of pepper. 3. Heat the olive oil in an oven-safe skillet over medium-high heat, and sear the tenderloin until browned on all sides, about 5 minutes total. 4. Transfer the skillet to the oven and roast for 12 to 15 minutes until the pork is cooked through, the juices run clear, and the internal temperature reaches 145°F. Transfer to a cutting board to rest for 5 minutes. 5. In a small bowl, combine the honey, vinegar, cooking wine, and ginger. In to the same skillet, pour the honey mixture and simmer for 1 minute. Add the mango and toss to coat. Transfer to a blender and purée until smooth. Season with the remaining ⅛ teaspoon of salt and ⅛ teaspoon of pepper. 6. Slice the pork into rounds and serve with the mango sauce.

Per Serving

Calories: 182 | fat: 4g | protein: 24 | carbs: 12g | sugars: 10g | fiber: 1g | sodium: 240mg

Dutch Oven Apple Pork Chops

Prep time: 20 minutes | Cook time: 20 minutes | Serves 4

4 bone-in pork loin chops, trimmed
¼ cup apple cider vinegar
1 teaspoon freshly ground black pepper
1 teaspoon ground cinnamon
1 teaspoon ground nutmeg
½ cup store-bought low-sodium chicken broth
3 celery stalks, cut into matchsticks
1 Candy Crisp apple, thinly sliced
1 small yellow onion, thinly sliced

1. Put the pork chops on a rimmed baking sheet. Season both sides with the vinegar, pepper, cinnamon, and nutmeg. 2. In a Dutch oven, bring the broth to a simmer over medium heat. 3. Add the pork chops and cook for 3 minutes, or until the exterior is browned. Transfer to a plate. 4. Add the celery, apple, and onion to the pot, making a bed. 5. Place the pork chops on top and cover. Cook for 10 to 15 minutes, taking care not to overcook. 6. Serve each pork chop with generous spoonfuls of apple, celery, and onion on the side.

Per Serving

Calorie: 298 | fat: 7g | protein: 40g | carbs: 18g | sugars: 12g | fiber: 2g | sodium: 122mg

Open-Faced Pulled Pork

Prep time: 15 minutes | Cook time: 1 hour 35minutes | Serves 2

2 tablespoons hoisin sauce
2 tablespoons tomato paste
2 tablespoons rice vinegar
1 tablespoon minced fresh ginger
2 teaspoons minced garlic
1 teaspoon chile-garlic sauce
¾ pound pork shoulder, trimmed of any visible fat, cut into 2-inch-square cubes
4 large romaine lettuce leaves

1. Preheat the oven to 300°F. 2. In a medium ovenproof pot with a tight-fitting lid, stir together the hoisin sauce, tomato paste, rice vinegar, ginger, garlic, and chile-garlic sauce. 3. Add the pork. Toss to coat. 4. Place the pot over medium heat. Bring to a simmer. Cover and carefully transfer the ovenproof pot to the preheated oven. Cook for 90 minutes. 5. Check the meat for doneness by inserting a fork into one of the chunks. If it goes in easily and the pork falls apart, the meat is done. If not, cook for another 30 minutes or so, until the meat passes the fork test. 6. Using a coarse strainer, strain the cooked pork into a fat separator. Shred the meat. Set aside. If you don't have a fat separator, remove the meat from the sauce and set aside. Let the sauce cool until any fat has risen to the top. With a spoon, remove as much fat as possible or use paper towels to blot it off. 7. In a small saucepan set over high heat, pour the defatted sauce. Bring to a boil, stirring frequently to prevent scorching. Cook for 2 to 3 minutes, or until thickened. 8. Add the shredded meat. Toss to coat with the sauce. Cook for 1 minute to reheat the meat. 9. Spoon equal amounts of pork into the romaine lettuce leaves and enjoy!

Per Serving

Calorie: 289 | fat: 11g | protein: 33g | carbs: 13g | sugars: 7g | fiber: 1g | sodium: 391mg

Steak Gyro Platter

Prep time: 30 minutes | Cook time: 8 to 10 minutes | Serves 4

1 pound (454 g) flank steak
1 teaspoon garlic powder
1 teaspoon ground cumin
½ teaspoon sea salt
½ teaspoon freshly ground black pepper
5 ounces (142 g) shredded romaine lettuce
½ cup crumbled feta cheese
½ cup peeled and diced cucumber
⅓ cup sliced red onion
¼ cup seeded and diced tomato
2 tablespoons pitted and sliced black olives
Tzatziki sauce, for serving

1. Pat the steak dry with paper towels. In a small bowl, combine the garlic powder, cumin, salt, and pepper. Sprinkle this mixture all over the steak, and allow the steak to rest at room temperature for 45 minutes. 2. Preheat the air fryer to 400°F (204°C). Place the steak in the air fryer basket and air fry for 4 minutes. Flip the steak and cook 4 to 6 minutes more, until an instant-read thermometer reads 120°F (49°C) at the thickest point for medium-rare (or as desired). Remove the steak from the air fryer and let it rest for 5 minutes. 3. Divide the romaine among plates. Top with the feta, cucumber, red onion, tomato, and olives.

Per Serving

Calorie: 229 | fat: 10g | protein: 28g | carbs: g5 | sugars: 2g | fiber: 2g | sodium: 559mg

Short Ribs with Chimichurri

Prep time: 30 minutes | Cook time: 13 minutes | Serves 4

1 pound (454 g) boneless short ribs
1½ teaspoons sea salt, divided
½ teaspoon freshly ground black pepper, divided
½ cup fresh parsley leaves
½ cup fresh cilantro leaves
1 teaspoon minced garlic
1 tablespoon freshly squeezed lemon juice
½ teaspoon ground cumin
¼ teaspoon red pepper flakes
2 tablespoons extra-virgin olive oil
Avocado oil spray

1. Pat the short ribs dry with paper towels. Sprinkle the ribs all over with 1 teaspoon salt and ¼ teaspoon black pepper. Let sit at room temperature for 45 minutes. 2. Meanwhile, place the parsley, cilantro, garlic, lemon juice, cumin, red pepper flakes, the remaining ½ teaspoon salt, and the remaining ¼ teaspoon black pepper in a blender or food processor. With the blender running, slowly drizzle in the olive oil. Blend for about 1 minute, until the mixture is smooth and well combined. 3. Set the air fryer to 400°F (204°C). Spray both sides of the ribs with oil. Place in the basket and air fry for 8 minutes. Flip and cook for another 5 minutes, until an instant-read thermometer reads 125°F (52°C) for medium-rare (or to your desired doneness). 4. Allow the meat to rest for 5 to 10 minutes, then slice. Serve warm with the chimichurri sauce.

Per Serving

Calorie: 251 | fat: 17g | protein: 25g | carbs: 1g | sugars: 0g | fiber: 1g | sodium: 651mg

Red Wine Pot Roast with Winter Vegetables

Prep time: 10 minutes | Cook time: 1 hour 35 minutes | Serves 6

One 3-pound boneless beef chuck roast or bottom round roast (see Note)
2 teaspoons fine sea salt
1 teaspoon freshly ground black pepper
1 tablespoon cold-pressed avocado oil
4 large shallots, quartered
4 garlic cloves, minced

1 cup dry red wine
2 tablespoons Dijon mustard
2 teaspoons chopped fresh rosemary
1 pound parsnips or turnips, cut into ½-inch pieces
1 pound carrots, cut into ½-inch pieces
4 celery stalks, cut into ½-inch pieces

1. Put the beef onto a plate, pat it dry with paper towels, and then season all over with the salt and pepper. 2. Select the Sauté setting on the Instant Pot and heat the oil for 2 minutes. Using tongs, lower the roast into the pot and sear for about 4 minutes, until browned on the first side. Flip the roast and sear for about 4 minutes more, until browned on the second side. Return the roast to the plate. 3. Add the shallots to the pot and sauté for about 2 minutes, until they begin to soften. Add the garlic and sauté for about 1 minute more. Stir in the wine, mustard, and rosemary, using a wooden spoon to nudge any browned bits from the bottom of the pot. Return the roast to the pot, then spoon some of the cooking liquid over the top. 4. Secure the lid and set the Pressure Release to Sealing. Press the Cancel button to reset the cooking program, then select the Meat/Stew setting and set the cooking time for 1 hour 5 minutes at high pressure. (The pot will take about 5 minutes to come up to pressure before the cooking program begins.) 5. When the cooking program ends, let the pressure release naturally for at least 15 minutes, then move the Pressure Release to Venting to release any remaining steam. Open the pot and, using tongs, carefully transfer the pot roast to a cutting board. Tent with aluminum foil to keep warm. 6. Add the parsnips, carrots, and celery to the pot. 7. Secure the lid and set the Pressure Release to Sealing. Press the Cancel button to reset the cooking program, then select the Pressure Cook or Manual setting and set the cooking time for 3 minutes at low pressure. (The pot will take about 10 minutes to come up to pressure before the cooking program begins.) 8. When the cooking program ends, perform a quick pressure release by moving the Pressure Release to Venting. Open the pot and, using a slotted spoon, transfer the vegetables to a serving dish. Wearing heat-resistant mitts, lift out the inner pot and pour the cooking liquid into a gravy boat or other serving vessel with a spout. (If you like, use a fat separator to remove the fat from the liquid before serving.) 9. If the roast was tied, snip the string and discard. Carve the roast against the grain into ½-inch-thick slices and arrange them on the dish with the vegetables. Pour some cooking liquid over the roast and serve, passing the remaining cooking liquid on the side.

Per Serving

Calorie: 448 | fat: 25g | protein: 26g | carbs: 26g | sugars: 7g | fiber: 6g | sodium: 945mg

Sage-Parmesan Pork Chops

Prep time: 30 minutes | Cook time: 25 minutes | Serves 2

Extra-virgin olive oil cooking spray
2 tablespoons coconut flour
¼ teaspoon salt
Pinch freshly ground black pepper
¼ cup almond meal
½ cup finely ground flaxseed meal

½ cup soy Parmesan cheese
1½ teaspoons rubbed sage
½ teaspoon grated lemon zest
2 (4-ounce) boneless pork chops
1 large egg, lightly beaten
1 tablespoon extra-virgin olive oil

1. Preheat the oven to 425°F. 2. Lightly coat a medium baking dish with cooking spray. 3. In a shallow dish, mix together the coconut flour, salt, and pepper. 4. In a second shallow dish, stir together the almond meal, flaxseed meal, soy Parmesan cheese, sage, and lemon zest. 5. Gently press one pork chop into the coconut flour mixture to coat. Shake off any excess. Dip into the beaten egg. Press into the almond meal mixture. Gently toss between your hands so any coating that hasn't stuck can fall away. Place the coated chop on a plate. Repeat the process with the remaining pork chop and coating ingredients. 6. In a large skillet set over medium heat, heat the olive oil. 7. Add the coated chops. Cook for about 4 minutes per side, or until browned. Transfer to the prepared baking dish. Place the dish in the preheated oven. Bake for 10 to 15 minutes, or until the juices run clear and an instant-read thermometer inserted into the middle of the pork reads 160°F.

Per Serving

Calorie: 520 | fat: 31g | protein: 45g | carbs: 14g | sugars: 1g | fiber: 6g | sodium: 403mg

Spiced Lamb Stew

Prep time: 20 minutes | Cook time: 2 hours | Serves 4

2 tablespoons extra-virgin olive oil
1½ pounds lamb shoulder, cut into 1-inch chunks
½ sweet onion, chopped
1 tablespoon grated fresh ginger
2 teaspoons minced garlic
1 teaspoon ground cinnamon

1 teaspoon ground cumin
¼ teaspoon ground cloves
2 sweet potatoes, peeled, diced
2 cups low-sodium beef broth
Sea salt
Freshly ground back pepper
2 teaspoons chopped fresh parsley, for garnish

1. Preheat the oven to 300°F. 2. Place a large ovenproof skillet over medium-high heat and add the olive oil. 3. Brown the lamb, stirring occasionally, for about 6 minutes. 4. Add the onion, ginger, garlic, cinnamon, cumin, and cloves, and sauté for 5 minutes. 5. Add the sweet potatoes and beef broth and bring the stew to a boil. 6. Cover the skillet and transfer the lamb to the oven. Braise, stirring occasionally, until the lamb is very tender, about 2 hours. 7. Remove the stew from the oven and season with salt and pepper. 8. Serve garnished with the parsley.

Per Serving

Calorie: 406 | fat: 21g | protein: 37g | carbs: 18g | sugars: 5g | fiber: 3g | sodium: 511mg

Creole Steak

Prep time: 5 minutes | Cook time: 1 hour 40 minutes | Serves 4

2 teaspoons extra-virgin olive oil
¼ cup chopped onion
¼ cup chopped green bell pepper
1 cup canned crushed tomatoes
½ teaspoon chili powder

¼ teaspoon celery seed
4 cloves garlic, finely chopped
¼ teaspoon salt
1 teaspoon cumin
1 pound lean boneless round steak

1. In a large skillet over medium heat, heat the oil. Add the onions and green pepper, and sauté until the onions are translucent (about 5 minutes). 2. Add the tomatoes, chili powder, celery seed, garlic, salt, and cumin; cover and let simmer over low heat for 20–25 minutes. This allows the flavors to blend. 3. Preheat the oven to 350 degrees. Trim all visible fat off the steak. 4. In a nonstick pan or a pan that has been sprayed with nonstick cooking spray, lightly brown the steak on each side. Transfer the steak to a 13-x-9-x-2-inch baking dish; pour the sauce over the steak, and cover. 5. Bake for 1¼ hours or until the steak is tender. Remove from the oven; slice the steak, and arrange on a serving platter. Spoon the sauce over the steak, and serve.

Per Serving

Calorie: 213 | fat: 10g | protein: 25g | carbs: 5g | sugars: 2g | fiber: 2g | sodium: 235mg

Slow-Cooked Simple Lamb and Vegetable Stew

Prep time: 10 minutes | Cook time: 3 to 10 hours | Serves 6

1 pound boneless lamb stew meat
1 pound turnips, peeled and chopped
1 fennel bupounds, trimmed and thinly sliced
10 ounces mushrooms, sliced
1 onion, diced
3 garlic cloves, minced
2 cups low-sodium chicken

broth
2 tablespoons tomato paste
¼ cup dry red wine (optional)
1 teaspoon chopped fresh thyme
½ teaspoon salt
¼ teaspoon freshly ground black pepper
Chopped fresh parsley, for garnish

1. In a slow cooker, combine the lamb, turnips, fennel, mushrooms, onion, garlic, chicken broth, tomato paste, red wine (if using), thyme, salt, and pepper. 2. Cover and cook on high for 3 hours or on low for 6 hours. When the meat is tender and falling apart, garnish with parsley and serve. 3. If you don't have a slow cooker, in a large pot, heat 2 teaspoons of olive oil over medium heat, and sear the lamb on all sides. Remove from the pot and set aside. Add the turnips, fennel, mushrooms, onion, and garlic to the pot, and cook for 3 to 4 minutes until the vegetables begin to soften. Add the chicken broth, tomato paste, red wine (if using), thyme, salt, pepper, and browned lamb. Bring to a boil, then reduce the heat to low. Simmer for 1½ to 2 hours until the meat is tender. Garnish with parsley and serve.

Per Serving

Calories: 303 | fat: 7g | protein: 32g | carbs: 27g | sugars: 7g | fiber: 4g | sodium: 310mg

Italian Beef Kebabs

Prep time: 25 minutes | Cook time: 10 minutes | Serves 2

2 garlic cloves, finely chopped
¼ cup balsamic vinegar
¼ cup water
2 tablespoons extra-virgin olive oil
1 tablespoon chopped fresh oregano leaves, or 1 teaspoon dried
1½ teaspoons chopped fresh marjoram leaves, or ½ teaspoon dried
1 teaspoon granulated stevia

1 (¾-pound, 1-inch-thick) beef bone-in sirloin, or round steak, fat removed, cut into 1-inch pieces
1 medium yellow squash, sliced
1 medium green bell pepper, cut into 1-inch squares
6 whole fresh button mushrooms
1 small red onion, cut into 1-inch squares

1. In a medium glass bowl, mix together the garlic, balsamic vinegar, water, olive oil, oregano, marjoram, and stevia. 2. Add the beef. Stir until coated. Cover and refrigerate, stirring occasionally, for at least 1 hour but no longer than 12 hours. 3. Preheat the oven to broil. 4. Remove the beef from the marinade, reserving the marinade. 5. Using 10-inch metal skewers, thread on 1 piece of beef, 1 piece of yellow squash, 1 piece of bell pepper, 1 mushroom, and 1 piece of onion, leaving ½ inch of space between each piece. Repeat with the remaining ingredients until all are used. Brush the kebabs with the reserved marinade. 6. Place the kebabs on a rack in the broiler pan. Place the pan under the preheated broiler about 3 inches from the heat. Broil for 6 to 8 minutes for medium-rare to medium doneness, turning and brushing with the marinade after 3 minutes. Discard any remaining marinade. 7. Enjoy this delightful meal on a stick!

Per Serving

Calorie: 494 | fat: 28g | protein: 42g | carbs: 19g | sugars: 11g | fiber: 4g | sodium: 114mg

Spinach and Provolone Steak Rolls

Prep time: 10 minutes | Cook time: 12 minutes | Makes 8 rolls

1 (1-pound / 454-g) flank steak, butterflied
8 (1-ounce / 28-g, ¼-inch-thick) deli slices provolone cheese

1 cup fresh spinach leaves
½ teaspoon salt
¼ teaspoon ground black pepper

1. Place steak on a large plate. Place provolone slices to cover steak, leaving 1-inch at the edges. Lay spinach leaves over cheese. Gently roll steak and tie with kitchen twine or secure with toothpicks. Carefully slice into eight pieces. Sprinkle each with salt and pepper. 2. Place rolls into ungreased air fryer basket, cut side up. Adjust the temperature to 400ºF (204ºC) and air fry for 12 minutes. Steak rolls will be browned and cheese will be melted when done and have an internal temperature of at least 150ºF (66ºC) for medium steak and 180ºF (82ºC) for well-done steak. Serve warm.

Per Serving

Calorie: 155 | fat: 8g | protein: 19g | carbs: 1g | sugars: 0g | fiber: 0g | sodium: 351mg

Roasted Beef with Peppercorn Sauce

Prep time: 10 minutes | Cook time:1hour | Serves 4

1½ pounds top rump beef roast
Sea salt
Freshly ground black pepper
3 teaspoons extra-virgin olive oil, divided
3 shallots, minced

2 teaspoons minced garlic
1 tablespoon green peppercorns
2 tablespoons dry sherry
2 tablespoons all-purpose flour
1 cup sodium-free beef broth

1. Heat the oven to 300°F. 2. Season the roast with salt and pepper. 3. Place a large skillet over medium-high heat and add 2 teaspoons of olive oil. 4. Brown the beef on all sides, about 10 minutes in total, and transfer the roast to a baking dish. 5. Roast until desired doneness, about 1½ hours for medium. When the roast has been in the oven for 1 hour, start the sauce. 6. In a medium saucepan over medium-high heat, sauté the shallots in the remaining 1 teaspoon of olive oil until translucent, about 4 minutes. 7. Stir in the garlic and peppercorns, and cook for another minute. Whisk in the sherry to deglaze the pan. 8. Whisk in the flour to form a thick paste, cooking for 1 minute and stirring constantly. 9. Pour in the beef broth and whisk until the sauce is thick and glossy, about 4 minutes. Season the sauce with salt and pepper. 10. Serve the beef with a generous spoonful of sauce.

Per Serving

Calorie: 272 | fat: 10g | protein: 40g | carbs: g | sugars: 0g | fiber: 0g | sodium: 331mg

Slow-Cooked Pork Burrito Bowls

Prep time: 15 minutes | Cook time: 8 to 10 hours | Serves 10

1 boneless pork shoulder (2 pounds), trimmed of excess fat
1 can (15 to 16 ounces) pinto beans, drained, rinsed
1 package (1 ounce) 40% less-sodium taco seasoning mix
1 can (4.5 ounces) diced green chiles, undrained

2 packages (7.6 ounces each) Spanish rice mix
5 cups water
1½ cups shredded Mexican cheese blend (6 ounces)
3 cups shredded lettuce
¾ cup chunky-style salsa

1. Spray 3- to 4-quart slow cooker with cooking spray. If pork comes in netting or is tied, remove netting or strings. Place pork in slow cooker. Pour beans around pork. Sprinkle taco seasoning mix over pork. Pour chiles over beans. 2. Cover; cook on Low heat setting 8 to 10 hours. 3. About 45 minutes before serving, in 3-quart saucepan, make rice mixes as directed on package, using water and omitting butter. 4. Remove pork from slow cooker; place on cutting board. Use 2 forks to pull pork into shreds. Return pork to slow cooker; gently stir to mix with beans. 5. To serve, spoon rice into each of 10 serving bowls; top each with pork mixture, cheese, lettuce and salsa.

Per Serving

Calories: 460 | fat: 17g | protein: 30g | carbs: 42g | sugars: 4g | fiber: 5g | sodium: 1030mg

Herb-Crusted Lamb Chops

Prep time: 10 minutes | Cook time: 5 minutes | Serves 2

1 large egg
2 cloves garlic, minced
¼ cup pork dust
¼ cup powdered Parmesan cheese
1 tablespoon chopped fresh oregano leaves
1 tablespoon chopped fresh rosemary leaves
1 teaspoon chopped fresh thyme leaves

½ teaspoon ground black pepper
4 (1-inch-thick) lamb chops
For Garnish/Serving (Optional):
Sprigs of fresh oregano
Sprigs of fresh rosemary
Sprigs of fresh thyme
Lavender flowers
Lemon slices

1. Spray the air fryer basket with avocado oil. Preheat the air fryer to 400ºF (204ºC). 2. Beat the egg in a shallow bowl, add the garlic, and stir well to combine. In another shallow bowl, mix together the pork dust, Parmesan, herbs, and pepper. 3. One at a time, dip the lamb chops into the egg mixture, shake off the excess egg, and then dredge them in the Parmesan mixture. Use your hands to coat the chops well in the Parmesan mixture and form a nice crust on all sides; if necessary, dip the chops again in both the egg and the Parmesan mixture. 4. Place the lamb chops in the air fryer basket, leaving space between them, and air fry for 5 minutes, or until the internal temperature reaches 145ºF (63ºC) for medium doneness. Allow to rest for 10 minutes before serving. 5. Garnish with sprigs of oregano, rosemary, and thyme, and lavender flowers, if desired. Serve with lemon slices, if desired. 6. Best served fresh. Store leftovers in an airtight container in the fridge for up to 4 days. Serve chilled over a salad, or reheat in a 350ºF (177ºC) air fryer for 3 minutes, or until heated through.

Per Serving

Calorie: 510 | fat: 42g | protein: 30g | carbs: 3g | sugars: 1g | fiber: 1g | sodium: 380mg

Easy Pot Roast and Vegetables

Prep time: 20 minutes | Cook time: 35 minutes | Serves 6

3–4 pound chuck roast, trimmed of fat and cut into serving-sized chunks
4 medium potatoes, cubed, unpeeled

4 medium carrots, sliced, or 1 pound baby carrots
2 celery ribs, sliced thin
1 envelope dry onion soup mix
3 cups water

1. Place the pot roast chunks and vegetables into the Instant Pot along with the potatoes, carrots and celery. 2. Mix together the onion soup mix and water and pour over the contents of the Instant Pot. 3. Secure the lid and make sure the vent is set to sealing. Set the Instant Pot to Manual mode for 35 minutes. Let pressure release naturally when cook time is up.

Per Serving

Calorie: 325 | fat: 8g | protein: 35g | carbs: 26g | sugars: 6g | fiber: 4g | sodium: 560mg

Steak Fajita Bake

Prep time: 10 minutes | Cook time: 15 minutes | Serves 4

1 green bell pepper	2 tablespoons avocado oil
1 yellow bell pepper	½ teaspoon ground cumin
1 red bell pepper	¼ teaspoon chili powder
1 small white onion	¼ teaspoon garlic powder
10 ounces sirloin steak, trimmed of visible fat	4 (6-inch) 100% whole-wheat tortillas

1. Preheat the oven to 400°F. 2. Cut the green bell pepper, yellow bell pepper, red bell pepper, onion, and steak into ½-inch-thick slices, and put them on a large baking sheet. 3. In a small bowl, combine the oil, cumin, chili powder, and garlic powder, then drizzle the mixture over the meat and vegetables to fully coat them. 4. Arrange the steak and vegetables in a single layer, and bake for 10 to 15 minutes, or until the steak is cooked through. 5. Divide the steak and vegetables equally between the tortillas.

Per Serving

Calorie: 360 | fat: 19g | protein: 20g | carbs: 27g | sugars: 4g | fiber: 6g | sodium: 257mg

Beef and Vegetable Shish Kabobs

Prep time: 15 minutes | Cook time: 20 minutes | Serves 8

2 teaspoons canola oil	1½ pounds boneless beef top sirloin steak, cut into 24 cubes
¼ cup red wine vinegar	
1 tablespoon light soy sauce	2 large bell peppers, red and green, cut into 1-inch pieces
4 garlic cloves, minced	
2 tablespoons freshly squeezed lemon juice	1 pound mushrooms, stemmed
⅛ teaspoon freshly ground black pepper	1 large tomato, cut into wedges
	1 medium onion, quartered

1. In a small bowl, combine the oil, vinegar, soy sauce, garlic, lemon juice, and pepper. Pour over the beef cubes, and let marinate in the refrigerator 3–4 hours or overnight. 2. Place 3 beef cubes on 8 metal or wooden skewers (remember to soak the wooden skewers in water before using), alternating with peppers, mushroom caps, tomato wedges, and onions. 3. Grill over medium heat, turning often and basting with marinade until the meat is cooked through. Arrange the skewers on a platter to serve.

Per Serving

Calorie: 211 | fat: 11g | protein: 20g | carbs: 7g | sugars: 4g | fiber: 2g | sodium: 82mg

Lamb Kofta Meatballs with Cucumber Quick-Pickled Salad

Prep time: 10 minutes | Cook time: 15 minutes | Serves 4

¼ cup red wine vinegar	½ red onion, finely chopped
Pinch red pepper flakes	1 pound ground lamb
1 teaspoon sea salt, divided	2 teaspoons ground coriander
2 cucumbers, peeled and chopped	1 teaspoon ground cumin
	3 garlic cloves, minced
1 tablespoon fresh mint, chopped	

1. Preheat the oven to 375°F. Line a rimmed baking sheet with parchment paper. 2. In a medium bowl, whisk together the vinegar, red pepper flakes, and ½ teaspoon of salt. Add the cucumbers and onion and toss to combine. Set aside. 3. In a large bowl, mix the lamb, coriander, cumin, garlic, mint, and remaining ½ teaspoon of salt. Form the mixture into 1-inch meatballs and place them on the prepared baking sheet. 4. Bake until the lamb reaches 140°F internally, about 15 minutes. 5. Serve with the salad on the side.

Per Serving

Calorie: 255 | fat: 14g | protein: 24g | carbs: 8g | sugars: 3g | fiber: 1g | sodium: 652mg

Lamb Chops with Cherry Glaze

Prep time: 10 minutes | Cook time: 20 minutes | Serves 4

4 (4-ounce) lamb chops	1 cup frozen cherries, thawed
1½ teaspoons chopped fresh rosemary	¼ cup dry red wine
	2 tablespoons orange juice
¼ teaspoon salt	1 teaspoon extra-virgin olive oil
¼ teaspoon freshly ground black pepper	

1. Season the lamb chops with the rosemary, salt, and pepper. 2. In a small saucepan over medium-low heat, combine the cherries, red wine, and orange juice, and simmer, stirring regularly, until the sauce thickens, 8 to 10 minutes. 3. Heat a large skillet over medium-high heat. When the pan is hot, add the olive oil to lightly coat the bottom. 4. Cook the lamb chops for 3 to 4 minutes on each side until well-browned yet medium rare. 5. Serve, topped with the cherry glaze.

Per Serving

Calories: 356 | fat: 27g | protein: 20g | carbs: 6g | sugars: 4g | fiber: 1g | sodium: 199mg

Sloppy Joes

Prep time: 10 minutes | Cook time: 15 minutes | Serves 4

1 pound 93% lean ground beef	2 tablespoons no-salt-added, no-sugar-added ketchup
½ medium yellow onion, chopped	
	2 tablespoons low-sodium Worcestershire sauce
1 medium red bell pepper, chopped	
	4 sandwich thins, 100% whole-wheat
1 (15-ounce) can no-salt-added tomato sauce	
	1 cup shredded cabbage

1. Heat a large skillet over medium heat. When hot, cook the beef, onion, and bell pepper for 7 to 10 minutes, stirring and breaking apart as needed. 2. Stir in the tomato sauce, ketchup, and Worcestershire sauce. Increase the heat to medium-high and simmer for 5 minutes. 3. Cut the sandwich thins in half so there is a top and a bottom. For each serving, place one-quarter of the filling and cabbage on the bottom half, then cover with the top half.

Per Serving

Calorie: 309 | fat: 8g | protein: 30g | carbs: 33g | sugars: 11g | fiber: 6g | sodium: 368mg

Pork Butt Roast

Prep time: 10 minutes | Cook time: 9 minutes | Serves 6 to 8

3–4-pound pork butt roast
2–3 tablespoons of your

favorite rub
2 cups water

1. Place pork in the inner pot of the Instant Pot. 2. Sprinkle in the rub all over the roast and add the water, being careful not to wash off the rub. 3. Secure the lid and set the vent to sealing. Cook for 9 minutes on the Manual setting. 4. Let the pressure release naturally.

Per Serving

Calories: 598 | fat: 40g | protein: 57g | carbs: 0g | sugars: 0g | fiber: 0g | sodium: 152mg

Beef Stew

Prep time: 30 minutes | Cook time: 1 hour 20 minutes | Serves 2

4 cups low-sodium beef broth, divided
3 tablespoons freshly squeezed lemon juice
2 teaspoons reduced-sodium soy sauce
2 teaspoons Worcestershire sauce
½ pound cubed beef stew meat
2 teaspoons extra-virgin olive oil
1 small onion, chopped
2 garlic cloves, minced

4 baby beets, tops removed, peeled, and cut into 1-inch cubes
1 cup chopped Brussels sprouts
2 medium carrots, sliced into 1-inch pieces
1 cup sliced baby portobello mushrooms
2 fresh thyme sprigs
⅛ teaspoon cayenne pepper
2 teaspoons cornstarch

1. In a large sealable plastic bag, combine 1 cup of beef broth, the lemon juice, soy sauce, and Worcestershire sauce. Add the beef. Seal the bag, turning to coat. Refrigerate for 8 hours, or overnight. 2. The next day, drain the beef and discard the marinade. 3. In a large saucepan set over medium heat, combine the olive oil and drained beef. Cook for 8 to 10 minutes, or until browned. Transfer the meat to a bowl and set aside. 4. To the same saucepan, add the onion. Sauté for 5 to 7 minutes, or until tender. 5. Add the garlic. Cook for 1 minute. 6. Add 2½ cups of beef broth. Return the meat to the pan. Increase the heat to high. Bring to a boil. Reduce the heat to low. Cover and simmer for 30 minutes. 7. Add the beets, Brussels sprouts, carrots, mushrooms, thyme, and cayenne pepper. Increase the heat to high. Return to a boil. Reduce the heat to low. Cover and simmer for 30 minutes, or until the vegetables and beef are tender. Remove and discard the thyme sprigs. 8. In a small bowl, whisk together the cornstarch and remaining ½ cup of beef broth until smooth. Gradually add to the stew, stirring to incorporate. Increase the heat to high. Bring to a boil again. Cook for 2 minutes, stirring, or until thickened.

Per Serving

Calorie: 428 | fat: 12g | protein: 40g | carbs: 44g | sugars: 18g | fiber: 10g | sodium: 499mg

Rosemary Roast Beef

Prep time: 30 minutes | Cook time: 30 to 35 minutes | Serves 8

1 (2-pound / 907-g) top round beef roast, tied with kitchen string
Sea salt and freshly ground black pepper, to taste

2 teaspoons minced garlic
2 tablespoons finely chopped fresh rosemary
¼ cup avocado oil

1. Season the roast generously with salt and pepper. 2. In a small bowl, whisk together the garlic, rosemary, and avocado oil. Rub this all over the roast. Cover loosely with aluminum foil or plastic wrap and refrigerate for at least 12 hours or up to 2 days. 3. Remove the roast from the refrigerator and allow to sit at room temperature for about 1 hour. 4. Set the air fryer to 325°F (163°C). Place the roast in the air fryer basket and roast for 15 minutes. Flip the roast and cook for 15 to 20 minutes more, until the meat is browned and an instant-read thermometer reads 120°F (49°C) at the thickest part (for medium-rare). 5. Transfer the meat to a cutting board, and let it rest for 15 minutes before thinly slicing and serving.

Per Serving

Calorie: 208 | fat: 12g | protein: 25g | carbs: 0g | sugars: 0g | fiber: 0g | sodium: 68mg

Pork Tenderloin Stir-Fry

Prep time: 5 minutes | Cook time: 20 minutes | Serves 6

1 tablespoon sesame oil
1-pound pork tenderloin, cut into thin strips
1 tablespoon oyster sauce (found in the Asian food section of the grocery store)
1 tablespoon cornstarch
½ cup low-sodium chicken broth

1 tablespoon light soy sauce
1 cup fresh snow peas, trimmed
1 cup broccoli florets
½ cup sliced water chestnuts, drained
1 cup diced red pepper
¼ cup sliced scallions

1. In a large skillet or wok, heat the oil. Stir-fry the pork until the strips are no longer pink. 2. In a measuring cup, combine the oyster sauce, cornstarch, chicken broth, and soy sauce. Add the sauce to the pork, and cook until the sauce thickens. 3. Add the vegetables, cover, and steam for 5 minutes. Serve.

Per Serving

Calorie: 149 | fat: 5g | protein: 18g | carbs: 8g | sugars: 3g | fiber: g | sodium: 174mg

Mediterranean Beef Steaks

Prep time: 20 minutes | Cook time: 20 minutes | Serves 4

2 tablespoons coconut aminos
3 heaping tablespoons fresh chives
2 tablespoons olive oil
3 tablespoons dry white wine
4 small-sized beef steaks

2 teaspoons smoked cayenne pepper
½ teaspoon dried basil
½ teaspoon dried rosemary
1 teaspoon freshly ground black pepper
1 teaspoon sea salt, or more to taste

1. Firstly, coat the steaks with the cayenne pepper, black pepper, salt, basil, and rosemary. 2. Drizzle the steaks with olive oil, white wine, and coconut aminos. 3. Finally, roast in the air fryer for 20 minutes at 340ºF (171ºC). Serve garnished with fresh chives. Bon appétit!

Per Serving

Calorie: 320 | fat: 17g | protein: 37g | carbs: g | sugars: 0g | fiber: 1g | sodium: 401mg

Butterflied Beef Eye Roast

Prep time: 10 minutes | Cook time: 40 minutes | Serves 12

3-pound lean beef eye roast
3 tablespoons extra-virgin olive oil
¼ cup water
½ cup red wine vinegar

3 garlic cloves, minced
½ teaspoon crushed red pepper
1 tablespoon chopped fresh thyme

1. Slice the roast down the middle, open it, and lay it flat in a shallow baking dish. 2. In a small bowl, combine the remaining ingredients, and pour the mixture over the roast. Cover, and let the meat marinate in the refrigerator for at least 12 hours, or up to 24 hours. Turn the roast occasionally. 3. Set the oven to broil. Remove the roast from the marinade, discard the marinade, and place the roast on a rack in the broiler pan. Broil the roast 5–7 inches from the heat, turning occasionally, for 20–25 minutes or until desired degree of doneness. 4. Remove from the oven, cover with foil, and let stand for 15–20 minutes before carving. Transfer to a serving platter, spoon any juices over the top, and serve.

Per Serving

Calorie: 191 | fat: 10g | protein: 24g | carbs: 0g | sugars: 0g | fiber: 0g | sodium: 98mg

Chapter 5 Poultry

Unstuffed Peppers with Ground Turkey and Quinoa   48

Teriyaki Chicken and Broccoli   48

One-Pan Chicken Dinner   48

Cilantro Lime Chicken Thighs   48

Thai Yellow Curry with Chicken Meatballs   49

Taco Stuffed Sweet Potatoes   49

Chicken Patties   49

Turkey Cabbage Soup   49

Mushroom-Sage Stuffed Turkey Breast   50

Coconut Chicken Curry   50

Tangy Barbecue Strawberry-Peach Chicken   50

Turkey–Butternut Squash Ragout   50

Turkey and Quinoa Caprese Casserole   51

Jerk Chicken Casserole   51

Greek Chicken Stuffed Peppers   51

Chicken with Mushroom Cream Sauce   51

Sautéed Chicken with Artichoke Hearts   52

Shredded Buffalo Chicken   52

Wine-Poached Chicken with Herbs and Vegetables   52

Peppered Chicken with Balsamic Kale   52

Baked Chicken Stuffed with Collard Greens   53

Teriyaki Turkey Meatballs   53

Lemony Chicken Thighs   53

Wild Rice and Turkey Casserole   53

Cheesy Stuffed Cabbage   54

Coconut Lime Chicken   54

Turkey Divan Casserole   54

Italian Chicken Thighs   54

Chicken with Lemon Caper Pan Sauce   55

Thanksgiving Turkey Breast   55

Herb-Roasted Turkey and Vegetables   55

Saffron-Spiced Chicken Breasts   55

Smoky Chicken Leg Quarters   56

Ginger Curry Chicken Kabobs   56

Orange Chicken Thighs with Bell Peppers   56

Fiber-Full Chicken Tostadas   56

Asian Mushroom-Chicken Soup   57

Fajita-Stuffed Chicken Breast   57

Cast Iron Hot Chicken   57

Speedy Chicken Cacciatore   57

Chicken Paprika   58

Orange Chicken   58

Chicken in Wine   58

Ginger Turmeric Chicken Thighs   58

Jerk Chicken Thighs   58

Tantalizing Jerked Chicken   59

Grain-Free Parmesan Chicken   59

Herbed Whole Turkey Breast   59

Unstuffed Peppers with Ground Turkey and Quinoa

Prep time: 0 minutes | Cook time: 35 minutes | Serves 8

2 tablespoons extra-virgin olive oil
1 yellow onion, diced
2 celery stalks, diced
2 garlic cloves, chopped
2 pounds 93 percent lean ground turkey
2 teaspoons Cajun seasoning blend (plus 1 teaspoon fine sea salt if using a salt-free blend)
½ teaspoon freshly ground black pepper
¼ teaspoon cayenne pepper
1 cup quinoa, rinsed

1 cup low-sodium chicken broth
One 14½-ounce can fire-roasted diced tomatoes and their liquid
3 red, orange, and/or yellow bell peppers, seeded and cut into 1-inch squares
1 green onion, white and green parts, thinly sliced
1½ tablespoons chopped fresh flat-leaf parsley
Hot sauce (such as Crystal or Frank's RedHot) for serving

1. Select the Sauté setting on the Instant Pot and heat the oil for 2 minutes. Add the onion, celery, and garlic and sauté for about 4 minutes, until the onion begins to soften. Add the turkey, Cajun seasoning, black pepper, and cayenne and sauté, using a wooden spoon or spatula to break up the meat as it cooks, for about 6 minutes, until cooked through and no streaks of pink remain. 2. Sprinkle the quinoa over the turkey in an even layer. Pour the broth and the diced tomatoes and their liquid over the quinoa, spreading the tomatoes on top. Sprinkle the bell peppers over the top in an even layer. 3. Secure the lid and set the Pressure Release to Sealing. Press the Cancel button to reset the cooking program, then select the Pressure Cook or Manual setting and set the cooking time for 8 minutes at high pressure. (The pot will take about 15 minutes to come up to pressure before the cooking program begins.) 4. When the cooking program ends, let the pressure release naturally for at least 15 minutes, then move the Pressure Release to Venting to release any remaining steam. Open the pot and sprinkle the green onion and parsley over the top in an even layer. 5. Spoon the unstuffed peppers into bowls, making sure to dig down to the bottom of the pot so each person gets an equal amount of peppers, quinoa, and meat. Serve hot, with hot sauce on the side.

Per Serving

Calories: 320 | fat: 14g | protein: 27g | carbs: 23g | sugars: 3g | fiber: 3g | sodium: 739mg

Teriyaki Chicken and Broccoli

Prep time: 5 minutes | Cook time: 20 minutes | Serves 4

For the sauce
½ cup water
2 tablespoons low-sodium soy sauce
2 tablespoons honey
1 tablespoon rice vinegar
¼ teaspoon garlic powder
Pinch ground ginger
1 tablespoon cornstarch

For the entrée
1 tablespoon sesame oil
4 (4-ounce) boneless, skinless chicken breasts, cut into bite-size cubes
1 (12-ounce) bag frozen broccoli
1 (12-ounce) bag frozen cauliflower rice

To make the sauce 1. In a small saucepan, whisk together the water, soy sauce, honey, rice vinegar, garlic powder, and ginger. Add the cornstarch and whisk until it is fully incorporated. 2. Over medium heat, bring the teriyaki sauce to a boil. Let the sauce boil for 1 minute to thicken. Remove the sauce from the heat and set aside. To make the entrée 1. Heat a large skillet over medium-low heat. When hot, add the oil and the chicken. Cook for 5 to 7 minutes, until the chicken is cooked through, stirring as needed. 2. Steam the broccoli and cauliflower rice in the microwave according to the package instructions. 3. Divide the cauliflower rice into four equal portions. Put one-quarter of the broccoli and chicken over each portion and top with the teriyaki sauce.

Per Serving

Calorie: 256 | fat: 7g | protein: 30g | carbs: 20g | sugars: 11g | fiber: 4g | sodium: 347mg

One-Pan Chicken Dinner

Prep time: 5 minutes | Cook time: 35 minutes | Serves 4

3 tablespoons extra-virgin olive oil
1 tablespoon red wine vinegar or apple cider vinegar
¼ teaspoon garlic powder
3 tablespoons Italian seasoning

4 (4-ounce) boneless, skinless chicken breasts
2 cups cubed sweet potatoes
20 Brussels sprouts, halved lengthwise

1. Preheat the oven to 400ºF. 2. In a large bowl, whisk together the oil, vinegar, garlic powder, and Italian seasoning. 3. Add the chicken, sweet potatoes, and Brussels sprouts, and coat thoroughly with the marinade. 4. Remove the ingredients from the marinade and arrange them on a baking sheet in a single layer. Roast for 15 minutes. 5. Remove the baking sheet from the oven, flip the chicken over, and bake for another 15 to 20 minutes.

Per Serving

Calorie: 346 | fat: 13g | protein: 30g | carbs: 26g | sugars: 6g | fiber: 7g | sodium: 575mg

Cilantro Lime Chicken Thighs

Prep time: 15 minutes | Cook time: 22 minutes | Serves 4

4 bone-in, skin-on chicken thighs
1 teaspoon baking powder
½ teaspoon garlic powder

2 teaspoons chili powder
1 teaspoon cumin
2 medium limes
¼ cup chopped fresh cilantro

1. Pat chicken thighs dry and sprinkle with baking powder. 2. In a small bowl, mix garlic powder, chili powder, and cumin and sprinkle evenly over thighs, gently rubbing on and under chicken skin. 3. Cut one lime in half and squeeze juice over thighs. Place chicken into the air fryer basket. 4. Adjust the temperature to 380ºF (193ºC) and roast for 22 minutes. 5. Cut other lime into four wedges for serving and garnish cooked chicken with wedges and cilantro.

Per Serving

Calorie: 445 | fat: 32g | protein: 32g | carbs: 6g | sugars: 1g | fiber: 2g | sodium: 198mg

Thai Yellow Curry with Chicken Meatballs

Prep time: 5 minutes | Cook time: 30 minutes | Serves 4

1 pound 95% lean ground chicken	into 1-inch lengths (or quartered if very large)
⅓ cup gluten-free panko (Japanese bread crumbs)	8 ounces zucchini, quartered lengthwise, then cut crosswise
1 egg white	into 1-inch lengths (or cut into
1 tablespoon coconut oil	halves, then thirds if large)
1 yellow onion, cut into 1-inch pieces	8 ounces cremini mushrooms, quartered
One 14-ounce can light coconut milk	Fresh Thai basil leaves for serving (optional)
3 tablespoons yellow curry paste	Fresno or jalapeño chile, thinly sliced, for serving (optional)
¾ cup water	1 lime, cut into wedges
8 ounces carrots, halved lengthwise, then cut crosswise	Cooked cauliflower "rice" for serving

1. In a medium bowl, combine the chicken, panko, and egg white and mix until evenly combined. Set aside. 2. Select the Sauté setting on the Instant Pot and heat the oil for 2 minutes. Add the onion and sauté for 5 minutes, until it begins to soften and brown. Add ½ cup of the coconut milk and the curry paste and sauté for 1 minute more, until bubbling and fragrant. Press the Cancel button to turn off the pot, then stir in the water. 3. Using a 1½-tablespoon cookie scoop, shape and drop meatballs into the pot in a single layer. 4. Secure the lid and set the Pressure Release to Sealing. Select the Pressure Cook or Manual setting and set the cooking time for 5 minutes at high pressure. (The pot will take about 5 minutes to come up to pressure before the cooking program begins.) 5. When the cooking program ends, perform a quick pressure release by moving the Pressure Release to Venting, or let the pressure release naturally. Open the pot and stir in the carrots, zucchini, mushrooms, and remaining 1¼ cups coconut milk. 6. Press the Cancel button to reset the cooking program, then select the Sauté setting. Bring the curry to a simmer (this will take about 2 minutes), then let cook, uncovered, for about 8 minutes, until the carrots are fork-tender. Press the Cancel button to turn off the pot. 7. Ladle the curry into bowls. Serve piping hot, topped with basil leaves and chile slices, if desired, and the lime wedges and cauliflower "rice" on the side.

Per Serving

Calories: 349 | fat: 15g | protein: 30g | carbs: 34g | sugars: 8g | fiber: 5g | sodium: 529mg

Taco Stuffed Sweet Potatoes

Prep time: 5 minutes | Cook time: 15 minutes | Serves 4

4 medium sweet potatoes	2 teaspoons ground cumin
2 tablespoons extra-virgin olive oil	1 teaspoon chili powder
1 pound 93% lean ground turkey	½ teaspoon salt
	½ teaspoon freshly ground black pepper

1. Pierce the potatoes with a fork, and microwave them on the potato setting, or for 10 minutes on high power. 2. Meanwhile, heat a medium skillet over medium heat. When hot, put the oil, turkey, cumin, chili powder, salt, and pepper into the skillet, stirring and breaking apart the meat, as needed. 3. Remove the potatoes from the microwave and halve them lengthwise. Depress the centers with a spoon, and fill each half with an equal amount of cooked turkey.

Per Serving

Calorie: 348 | fat: 17g | protein: 24g | carbs: 27g | sugars: 6g | fiber: 4g | sodium: 462mg

Chicken Patties

Prep time: 15 minutes | Cook time: 12 minutes | Serves 4

1 pound (454 g) ground chicken thigh meat	½ teaspoon garlic powder
½ cup shredded Mozzarella cheese	¼ teaspoon onion powder
	1 large egg
1 teaspoon dried parsley	2 ounces (57 g) pork rinds, finely ground

1. In a large bowl, mix ground chicken, Mozzarella, parsley, garlic powder, and onion powder. Form into four patties. 2. Place patties in the freezer for 15 to 20 minutes until they begin to firm up. 3. Whisk egg in a medium bowl. Place the ground pork rinds into a large bowl. 4. Dip each chicken patty into the egg and then press into pork rinds to fully coat. Place patties into the air fryer basket. 5. Adjust the temperature to 360ºF (182ºC) and air fry for 12 minutes. 6. Patties will be firm and cooked to an internal temperature of 165ºF (74ºC) when done. Serve immediately.

Per Serving

Calorie: 265 | fat: 15g | protein: 29g | carbs: 1g | sugars: 0g | fiber: 0g | sodium: 285mg

Turkey Cabbage Soup

Prep time: 15 minutes | Cook time: 30 minutes | Serves 4

1 tablespoon extra-virgin olive oil	1 sweet potato, peeled, diced
1 sweet onion, chopped	8 cups chicken or turkey broth
2 celery stalks, chopped	2 bay leaves
2 teaspoons minced fresh garlic	1 cup chopped cooked turkey
	2 teaspoons chopped fresh thyme
4 cups finely shredded green cabbage	Sea salt
	Freshly ground black pepper

1. Place a large saucepan over medium-high heat and add the olive oil. 2. Sauté the onion, celery, and garlic until softened and translucent, about 3 minutes. 3. Add the cabbage and sweet potato and sauté for 3 minutes. 4. Stir in the chicken broth and bay leaves and bring the soup to a boil. 5. Reduce the heat to low and simmer until the vegetables are tender, about 20 minutes. 6. Add the turkey and thyme and simmer until the turkey is heated through, about 4 minutes. 7. Remove the bay leaves and season the soup with salt and pepper.

Per Serving

Calorie: 444 | fat: 14g | protein: 38g | carbs: 42g | sugars: 17g | fiber: 7g | sodium: 427mg

Mushroom-Sage Stuffed Turkey Breast

Prep time: 10 minutes | Cook time: 1 hour 5 minutes | Serves 8

2 tablespoons extra-virgin olive oil, divided
8 ounces brown mushrooms, finely chopped
2 garlic cloves, minced
½ teaspoon salt, divided
¼ teaspoon freshly ground

black pepper, divided
2 tablespoons chopped fresh sage
1 boneless, skinless turkey breast (about 3 pounds), butterflied

1. Preheat the oven to 375°F. 2. In a large skillet, heat 1 tablespoon of oil over medium heat. Add the mushrooms and cook for 4 to 5 minutes, stirring regularly, until most of the liquid has evaporated from the pan. Add the garlic, ¼ teaspoon of salt, and ⅛ teaspoon of pepper, and continue to cook for an additional minute. Add the sage to the pan, cook for 1 minute, and remove the pan from the heat. 3. On a clean work surface, lay the turkey breast flat. Use a kitchen mallet to pound the breast to an even 1-inch thickness throughout. 4. Spread the mushroom-sage mixture on the turkey breast, leaving a 1-inch border around the edges. Roll the breast tightly into a log. 5. Using kitchen twine, tie the breast two or three times around to hold it together. Rub the remaining 1 tablespoon of oil over the turkey breast. Season with the remaining ¼ teaspoon of salt and ⅛ teaspoon of pepper. 6. Transfer to a roasting pan and roast for 50 to 60 minutes, until the juices run clear, the meat is cooked through, and the internal temperature reaches 180°F. 7. Let rest for 5 minutes. Cut off the twine, slice, and serve.

Per Serving

Calories: 232 | fat: 6g | protein: 41g | carbs: 2g | sugars: 0g | fiber: 0g | sodium: 320mg

Coconut Chicken Curry

Prep time: 15 minutes | Cook time: 35 minutes | Serves 4

2 teaspoons extra-virgin olive oil
3 (5-ounce) boneless, skinless chicken breasts, cut into 1-inch chunks
1 tablespoon grated fresh ginger
1 tablespoon minced garlic

2 tablespoons curry powder
2 cups low-sodium chicken broth
1 cup canned coconut milk
1 carrot, peeled and diced
1 sweet potato, diced
2 tablespoons chopped fresh cilantro

1. Place a large saucepan over medium-high heat and add the oil. 2. Sauté the chicken until lightly browned and almost cooked through, about 10 minutes. 3. Add the ginger, garlic, and curry powder, and sauté until fragrant, about 3 minutes. 4. Stir in the chicken broth, coconut milk, carrot, and sweet potato and bring the mixture to a boil. 5. Reduce the heat to low and simmer, stirring occasionally, until the vegetables and chicken are tender, about 20 minutes. 6. Stir in the cilantro and serve.

Per Serving

Calorie: 327 | fat: 18g | protein: 29g | carbs: 14g | sugars: 2g | fiber: 3g | sodium: 122mg

Tangy Barbecue Strawberry-Peach Chicken

Prep time: 20 minutes | Cook time: 40 minutes | Serves 4

For the barbecue sauce
1 cup frozen peaches
1 cup frozen strawberries
¼ cup tomato purée
½ cup white vinegar
1 tablespoon yellow mustard
1 teaspoon mustard seeds
1 teaspoon turmeric
1 teaspoon sweet paprika

1 teaspoon garlic powder
½ teaspoon cayenne pepper
½ teaspoon onion powder
½ teaspoon freshly ground black pepper
1 teaspoon celery seeds
For the chicken
4 boneless, skinless chicken thighs

To make the barbecue sauce 1. In a stockpot, combine the peaches, strawberries, tomato purée, vinegar, mustard, mustard seeds, turmeric, paprika, garlic powder, cayenne, onion powder, black pepper, and celery seeds. Cook over low heat for 15 minutes, or until the flavors come together. 2. Remove the sauce from the heat, and let cool for 5 minutes. 3. Transfer the sauce to a blender, and purée until smooth. To make the chicken 1. Preheat the oven to 350°F. 2. Put the chicken in a medium bowl. Coat well with ½ cup of barbecue sauce. 3. Place the chicken on a rimmed baking sheet. 4. Place the baking sheet on the middle rack of the oven, and bake for about 20 minutes (depending on the thickness of thighs), or until the juices run clear. 5. Brush the chicken with additional sauce, return to the oven, and broil on high for 3 to 5 minutes, or until a light crust forms. 6. Serve.

Per Serving

Calorie: 389 | fat: 8g | protein: 63g | carbs: 13g | sugars: 7g | fiber: 3g | sodium: 175mg

Turkey–Butternut Squash Ragout

Prep time: 15 minutes | Cook time: 7 to 8 hours | Serves 4

1½ pounds turkey thighs (about 2 medium), skin removed
1 small butternut squash (about 2 pounds), peeled, seeded, cut into 1½-inch pieces (3 cups)
1 medium onion, cut in half, then cut into slices

1 can (16 ounces) baked beans, undrained
1 can (14.5 ounces) diced tomatoes with Italian herbs, undrained
2 tablespoons chopped fresh parsley

1. Spray 3- to 4-quart slow cooker with cooking spray. In slow cooker, mix all ingredients except parsley. 2. Cover; cook on Low heat setting 7 to 8 hours. 3. Transfer turkey from slow cooker to cutting board. Remove meat from bones; discard bones. Return turkey to slow cooker and stir to reheat. Just before serving, sprinkle with parsley.

Per Serving

Calories: 410 | fat: 6g | protein: 46g | carbs: 41g | sugars: 16g | fiber: 7g | sodium: 690mg

Turkey and Quinoa Caprese Casserole

Prep time: 10 minutes | Cook time: 35 minutes | Serves 8

⅔ cup quinoa
1⅓ cups water
Nonstick cooking spray
2 teaspoons extra-virgin olive oil
1 pound lean ground turkey
¼ cup chopped red onion
½ teaspoon salt
1 (15-ounce can) fire-roasted tomatoes, drained

4 cups spinach leaves, finely sliced
3 garlic cloves, minced
¼ cup sliced fresh basil
¼ cup chicken or vegetable broth
2 large ripe tomatoes, sliced
4 ounces mozzarella cheese, thinly sliced

1. In a small pot, combine the quinoa and water. Bring to a boil, reduce the heat, cover, and simmer for 10 minutes. Turn off the heat, and let the quinoa sit for 5 minutes to absorb any remaining water. 2. Preheat the oven to 400°F. Spray a baking dish with nonstick cooking spray. 3. In a large skillet, heat the oil over medium heat. Add the turkey, onion, and salt. Cook until the turkey is cooked through and crumbled. 4. Add the tomatoes, spinach, garlic, and basil. Stir in the broth and cooked quinoa. Transfer the mixture to the prepared baking dish. Arrange the tomato and cheese slices on top. 5. Bake for 15 minutes until the cheese is melted and the tomatoes are softened. Serve.

Per Serving

Calories: 218 | fat: 9g | protein: 18g | carbs: 17g | sugars: 3g | fiber: 3g | sodium: 340mg

Jerk Chicken Casserole

Prep time: 15 minutes | Cook time: 45 minutes | Serves 6

1¼ teaspoons salt
½ teaspoon pumpkin pie spice
¾ teaspoon ground allspice
¾ teaspoon dried thyme leaves
¼ teaspoon ground red pepper (cayenne)
6 boneless skinless chicken thighs
1 tablespoon vegetable oil

1 can (15 ounces) black beans, drained, rinsed
1 large sweet potato (1 pound), peeled, cubed (3 cups)
¼ cup honey
¼ cup lime juice
2 teaspoons cornstarch
2 tablespoons sliced green onions (2 medium)

1. Heat oven to 375°F. Spray 8-inch square (2-quart) glass baking dish with cooking spray. In small bowl, mix salt, pumpkin pie spice, allspice, thyme and red pepper. Rub mixture on all sides of chicken. In 12-inch nonstick skillet, heat oil over medium-high heat. Cook chicken in oil 2 to 3 minutes per side, until brown. 2. In baking dish, layer beans and sweet potato. Top with browned chicken. In small bowl, mix honey, lime juice and cornstarch; add to skillet. Heat to boiling, stirring constantly. Pour over chicken in baking dish. 3. Bake 35 to 45 minutes or until juice of chicken is clear when center of thickest part is cut (165°F) and sweet potatoes are fork-tender. Sprinkle with green onions.

Per Serving

Calories: 330 | fat: 8g | protein: 21g | carbs: 43g | sugars: 16g | fiber: 9g | sodium: 550mg

Greek Chicken Stuffed Peppers

Prep time: 5 minutes | Cook time: 30 minutes | Serves 4

2 large red bell peppers
2 teaspoons extra-virgin olive oil, divided
½ cup uncooked brown rice or quinoa
4 (4-ounce) boneless, skinless

chicken breasts
¼ teaspoon garlic powder
¼ teaspoon onion powder
⅛ teaspoon dried thyme
½ teaspoon dried oregano
½ cup crumbled feta

1. Cut the bell peppers in half and remove the seeds. 2. In a large skillet, heat 1 teaspoon of olive oil over low heat. When hot, place the bell pepper halves cut-side up in the skillet. Cover and cook for 20 minutes. 3. Cook the rice according to the package instructions. 4. Meanwhile, cut the chicken into 1-inch pieces. 5. In a medium skillet, heat the remaining 1 teaspoon of olive oil over medium-low heat. When hot, add the chicken. 6. Season the chicken with the garlic powder, onion powder, thyme, and oregano. 7. Cook for 5 minutes, stirring occasionally, until cooked through. 8. In a large bowl, combine the cooked rice and chicken. Scoop one-quarter of the chicken and rice mixture into each pepper half, cover, and cook for 10 minutes over low heat. 9. Top each pepper half with 2 tablespoons of crumbled feta.

Per Serving

Calorie: 311 | fat: 11g | protein: 32g | carbs: 20g | sugars: 4g | fiber: 3g | sodium: 228mg

Chicken with Mushroom Cream Sauce

Prep time: 5 minutes | Cook time: 20 minutes | Serves 8

1 tablespoon extra-virgin olive oil
Eight 3-ounce boneless, skinless chicken breast halves
½ cup sliced mushrooms
3 tablespoons flour
½ cup low-sodium chicken

broth
¾ cup white wine
2 teaspoons lemon zest
½ teaspoons lemon pepper
1 cup plain fat-free Greek yogurt
Parsley sprigs

1. In a large nonstick skillet, heat the oil; add the chicken and cook for 5 minutes on each side. Remove the chicken, and keep warm. Add the mushrooms to the skillet, and cook until tender. 2. In a small bowl, whisk the flour with the broth and wine. Stir the mixture into the skillet, and add the lemon zest and pepper. Cook until thickened and bubbly. 3. Return the chicken to the skillet, and cook until the chicken is no longer pink. Transfer the chicken to a platter. Stir the yogurt into the skillet and heat thoroughly. Pour the sauce over the chicken, and garnish with parsley.

Per Serving

Calorie: 166 | fat: 4g | protein: 22g | carbs: 6g | sugars: 3g | fiber: 0g | sodium: 68mg

Sautéed Chicken with Artichoke Hearts

Prep time: 5 minutes | Cook time: 20 minutes | Serves 4

Nonstick cooking spray
Three 8-ounce boneless, skinless chicken breasts, halved
½ cup low-sodium chicken stock
¼ cup dry white wine
Two 8-ounce cans artichoke hearts, packed in water, drained and quartered
1 medium onion, diced
1 medium green bell pepper, chopped
2 tablespoons minced fresh tarragon or mint
¼ teaspoon white pepper
2 teaspoons cornstarch
1 tablespoon cold water
2 medium tomatoes, cut into wedges

1. Coat a large skillet with nonstick cooking spray; place over medium heat until hot. Add the chicken, and sauté until lightly browned, about 3–4 minutes per side. 2. Add the chicken stock, wine, artichokes, onion, green pepper, tarragon or mint, and white pepper; stir well. Bring to a boil, cover, reduce heat, and let simmer for 10–15 minutes or until the chicken is no longer pink and the vegetables are just tender. 3. In a small bowl, combine the cornstarch and water; add to the chicken mixture along with the tomato wedges, stirring until the mixture has thickened. Remove from the heat, and serve.

Per Serving

Calorie: 310 | fat: 5g | protein: 44g | carbs: 21g | sugars: 5g | fiber: 8g | sodium: 199mg

Shredded Buffalo Chicken

Prep time: 10 minutes | Cook time: 20 minutes | Serves 8

2 tablespoons avocado oil
½ cup finely chopped onion
1 celery stalk, finely chopped
1 large carrot, chopped
⅓ cup mild hot sauce (such as Frank's RedHot)
½ tablespoon apple cider vinegar
¼ teaspoon garlic powder
2 bone-in, skin-on chicken breasts (about 2 pounds)

1. Set the electric pressure cooker to the Sauté setting. When the pot is hot, pour in the avocado oil. 2. Sauté the onion, celery, and carrot for 3 to 5 minutes or until the onion begins to soften. Hit Cancel. 3. Stir in the hot sauce, vinegar, and garlic powder. Place the chicken breasts in the sauce, meat-side down. 4. Close and lock the lid of the pressure cooker. Set the valve to sealing. 5. Cook on high pressure for 20 minutes. 6. When cooking is complete, hit Cancel and quick release the pressure. Once the pin drops, unlock and remove the lid. 7. Using tongs, transfer the chicken breasts to a cutting board. When the chicken is cool enough to handle, remove the skin, shred the chicken and return it to the pot. Let the chicken soak in the sauce for at least 5 minutes. 8. Serve immediately.

Per Serving

Calorie: 235 | fat: 14g | protein: 24g | carbs: 2g | sugars: 1g | fiber: 1g | sodium: 142mg

Wine-Poached Chicken with Herbs and Vegetables

Prep time: 5 minutes | Cook time: 1 hour | Serves 8

4 quarts low-sodium chicken broth
2 cups dry white wine
4 large bay leaves
4 sprigs fresh thyme
¼ teaspoon freshly ground black pepper
4-pound chicken, giblets removed, washed and patted
dry
½ pound carrots, peeled and julienned
½ pound turnips, peeled and julienned
½ pound parsnips, peeled and julienned
4 small leeks, washed and trimmed

1. In a large stockpot, combine the broth, wine, bay leaves, thyme, dash salt (optional), and pepper. Let simmer over medium heat while you prepare the chicken. 2. Stuff the cavity with ⅓ each of the carrots, turnips, and parsnips; then truss. Add the stuffed chicken to the stockpot, and poach, covered, over low heat for 30 minutes. 3. Add the remaining vegetables with the leeks, and continue to simmer for 25–30 minutes, or until juices run clear when the chicken is pierced with a fork. 4. Remove the chicken and vegetables to a serving platter. Carve the chicken, remove the skin, and surround the sliced meat with poached vegetables to serve.

Per Serving

Calorie: 476 | fat: 13g | protein: 57g | carbs: 24g | sugars: 6g | fiber: 4g | sodium: 387mg

Peppered Chicken with Balsamic Kale

Prep time: 5 minutes | Cook time: 15 minutes | Serves 4

4 (4-ounce) boneless, skinless chicken breasts
¼ teaspoon salt
1 tablespoon freshly ground black pepper
2 tablespoons unsalted butter
1 tablespoon extra-virgin olive
oil
8 cups stemmed and roughly chopped kale, loosely packed (about 2 bunches)
½ cup balsamic vinegar
20 cherry tomatoes, halved

1. Season both sides of the chicken breasts with the salt and pepper. 2. Heat a large skillet over medium heat. When hot, heat the butter and oil. Add the chicken and cook for 8 to 10 minutes, flipping halfway through. When cooked all the way through, remove the chicken from the skillet and set aside. 3. Increase the heat to medium-high. Put the kale in the skillet and cook for 3 minutes, stirring every minute. 4. Add the vinegar and the tomatoes and cook for another 3 to 5 minutes. 5. Divide the kale and tomato mixture into four equal portions, and top each portion with 1 chicken breast.

Per Serving

calorie: 383 | fat: 12g | protein: 34g | carbs: 38g | sugars: 25g | fiber: 11g | sodium: 256mg

Baked Chicken Stuffed with Collard Greens

Prep time: 10 minutes | Cook time: 30 minutes | Serves 4

For the gravy
2½ cups store-bought low-sodium chicken broth, divided
4 tablespoons whole-wheat flour, divided
1 medium yellow onion, chopped
½ bunch fresh thyme, roughly chopped
2 garlic cloves, minced
1 bay leaf
½ teaspoon celery seeds
1 teaspoon Worcestershire sauce
Freshly ground black pepper

For the chicken
2 boneless, skinless chicken breasts
Juice of 1 lime
1 teaspoon sweet paprika
½ teaspoon onion powder
½ teaspoon garlic powder
2 medium tomatoes, chopped
1 bunch collard greens, center stem removed, cut into 1-inch ribbons
¼ cup chicken broth (optional)
Generous pinch red pepper flakes

To make the gravy 1. In a shallow stockpot, combine ½ cup of broth and 1 tablespoon of flour and cook over medium-low heat, whisking until the flour is dissolved. Continue to add 1 cup of broth and the remaining 3 tablespoons of flour in increments until a thick sauce is formed. 2. Add the onion, thyme, garlic, bay leaf, and ½ cup of broth, stirring well. To make the chicken 1. Cut a slit in each chicken breast deep enough for stuffing along its entire length. 2. In a small mixing bowl, massage the chicken all over with the lime juice, paprika, onion powder, and garlic powder. 3. In an electric pressure cooker, combine the tomatoes and collard greens. If the mixture looks dry, add the chicken broth. 4. Close and lock the lid, and set the pressure valve to sealing. 5. Select the Manual/Pressure Cook setting, and cook for 2 minutes. 6. Once cooking is complete, quick-release the pressure. Carefully remove the lid. 7. Using tongs or a slotted spoon, remove the greens while leaving the tomatoes behind. 8. Stuff the chicken breasts with the greens. Lay on the bed of tomatoes in the pressure cooker, with the side with greens facing up. 9. Spoon half of the gravy over the stuffed chicken. 10. Close and lock the lid, and set the pressure valve to sealing. 11. Select the Manual/Pressure Cook setting, and cook for 10 minutes. 12. Once cooking is complete, quick-release the pressure. Carefully remove the lid. 13. Remove the chicken and tomatoes from pressure cooker, and transfer to a serving dish. Season with the red pepper flakes.

Per Serving

Calorie: 301 | fat: 6g | protein: 41g | carbs: 24g | sugars: 4g | fiber: 9g | sodium: 155mg

Teriyaki Turkey Meatballs

Prep time: 20 minutes | Cook time: 20 minutes | Serves 6

1 pound lean ground turkey
¼ cup finely chopped scallions, both white and green parts
1 egg
2 garlic cloves, minced

1 teaspoon grated fresh ginger
2 tablespoons reduced-sodium tamari or gluten-free soy sauce
1 tablespoon honey
2 teaspoons mirin
1 teaspoon toasted sesame oil

1. Preheat the oven to 400°F. Line a baking sheet with parchment paper. 2. In a large mixing bowl, combine the turkey, scallions, egg, garlic, ginger, tamari, honey, mirin, and sesame oil. Mix well. 3. Using your hands, form the meat mixture into balls about the size of a tablespoon. Arrange on the prepared baking sheet. 4. Bake for 10 minutes, flip with a spatula, and continue baking for an additional 10 minutes until the meatballs are cooked through.

Per Serving

Calories: 153 | fat: 8g | protein: 16g | carbs: 5g | sugars: 4g | fiber: 0g | sodium: 270mg

Lemony Chicken Thighs

Prep time: 15 minutes | Cook time: 15 minutes | Serves 3 to 5

1 cup low-sodium chicken bone broth
5 frozen bone-in chicken thighs
1 small onion, diced
5–6 cloves garlic, diced
Juice of 1 lemon
2 tablespoons margarine,

melted
½ teaspoon salt
¼ teaspoon black pepper
1 teaspoon True Lemon Lemon Pepper seasoning
1 teaspoon parsley flakes
¼ teaspoon oregano
Rind of 1 lemon

1. Add the chicken bone broth into the inner pot of the Instant Pot. 2. Add the chicken thighs. 3. Add the onion and garlic. 4. Pour the fresh lemon juice in with the melted margarine. 5. Add the seasonings. 6. Lock the lid, make sure the vent is at sealing, then press the Poultry button. Set to 15 minutes. 7. When cook time is up, let the pressure naturally release for 3–5 minutes, then manually release the rest. 8. You can place these under the broiler for 2–3 minutes to brown. 9. Plate up and pour some of the sauce over top with fresh grated lemon rind.

Per Serving

Calories: 329 | fat: 24g | protein: 26g | carbs: 3g | sugars: 1g | fiber: 0g | sodium: 407mg

Wild Rice and Turkey Casserole

Prep time: 10 minutes | Cook time: 55 minutes | Serves 6

2 cups cut-up cooked turkey or chicken
2¼ cups boiling water
⅓ cup fat-free (skim) milk
4 medium green onions, sliced (¼ cup)
1 can (10.75 ounces)

condensed 98% fat-free cream of mushroom soup
1 package (6 ounces) original long-grain and wild rice mix
Additional green onions, if desired

1. Heat oven to 350°F. In ungreased 2-quart casserole, mix all ingredients, including seasoning packet from rice mix. 2. Cover; bake 45 to 50 minutes or until rice is tender. Uncover; bake 10 to 15 minutes longer or until liquid is absorbed. Sprinkle with additional green onions.

Per Serving

Calories: 220 | fat: 4.5g | protein: 17g | carbs: 27g | sugars: 2g | fiber: 1g | sodium: 740mg

Cheesy Stuffed Cabbage

Prep time: 30 minutes | Cook time: 18 minutes | Serves 6 to 8

1–2 heads savoy cabbage
1 pound ground turkey
1 egg
1 cup reduced-fat shredded cheddar cheese
2 tablespoons evaporated skim milk
¼ cup reduced-fat shredded Parmesan cheese
¼ cup reduced-fat shredded mozzarella cheese
¼ cup finely diced onion
¼ cup finely diced bell pepper
¼ cup finely diced mushrooms
1 teaspoon salt
½ teaspoon black pepper
1 teaspoon garlic powder
6 basil leaves, fresh and cut chiffonade
1 tablespoon fresh parsley, chopped
1 quart of your favorite pasta sauce

1. Remove the core from the cabbages. 2. Boil pot of water and place 1 head at a time into the water for approximately 10 minutes. 3. Allow cabbage to cool slightly. Once cooled, remove the leaves carefully and set aside. You'll need about 15 or 16. 4. Mix together the meat and all remaining ingredients except the pasta sauce. 5. One leaf at a time, put a heaping tablespoon of meat mixture in the center. 6. Tuck the sides in and then roll tightly. 7. Add ½ cup sauce to the bottom of the inner pot of the Instant Pot. 8. Place the rolls, fold-side down, into the pot and layer them, putting a touch of sauce between each layer and finally on top. (You may want to cook the rolls in two batches.) 9. Lock lid and make sure vent is at sealing. Set timer on 18 minutes on Manual at high pressure, then manually release the pressure when cook time is over.

Per Serving

Calories: 199| fat: 8g | protein: 2mg | carbs: 14g | sugars: 7g | fiber: 3g | sodium: 678mg

Coconut Lime Chicken

Prep time: 5 minutes | Cook time: 15 minutes | Serves 4

1 tablespoon coconut oil
4 (4-ounce) boneless, skinless chicken breasts
½ teaspoon salt
1 red bell pepper, cut into ¼-inch-thick slices
16 asparagus spears, bottom ends trimmed
1 cup unsweetened coconut milk
2 tablespoons freshly squeezed lime juice
½ teaspoon garlic powder
¼ teaspoon red pepper flakes
¼ cup chopped fresh cilantro

1. In a large skillet, heat the oil over medium-low heat. When hot, add the chicken. 2. Season the chicken with the salt. Cook for 5 minutes, then flip. 3. Push the chicken to the side of the skillet, and add the bell pepper and asparagus. Cook, covered, for 5 minutes. 4. Meanwhile, in a small bowl, whisk together the coconut milk, lime juice, garlic powder, and red pepper flakes. 5. Add the coconut milk mixture to the skillet, and boil over high heat for 2 to 3 minutes. 6. Top with the cilantro.

Per Serving

Calorie: 319 | fat: 21g | protein: 28g | carbs: 7g | sugars: 4g | fiber: 2g | sodium: 353mg

Turkey Divan Casserole

Prep time: 10 minutes | Cook time: 50 minutes | Serves 6

Nonstick cooking spray
3 teaspoons extra-virgin olive oil, divided
1 pound turkey cutlets
Pinch salt
¼ teaspoon freshly ground black pepper, divided
¼ cup chopped onion
2 garlic cloves, minced
2 tablespoons whole-wheat flour
1 cup unsweetened plain almond milk
1 cup low-sodium chicken broth
½ cup shredded Swiss cheese, divided
½ teaspoon dried thyme
4 cups chopped broccoli
¼ cup coarsely ground almonds

1. Preheat the oven to 375°F. Spray a baking dish with nonstick cooking spray. 2. In a skillet, heat 1 teaspoon of oil over medium heat. Season the turkey with the salt and ⅛ teaspoon of pepper. Sauté the turkey cutlets for 5 to 7 minutes on each side until cooked through. Transfer to a cutting board, cool briefly, and cut into bite-size pieces. 3. In the same pan, heat the remaining 2 teaspoons of oil over medium-high heat. Sauté the onion for 3 minutes until it begins to soften. Add the garlic and continue cooking for another minute. 4. Stir in the flour and mix well. Whisk in the almond milk, broth, and remaining ⅛ teaspoon of pepper, and continue whisking until smooth. Add ¼ cup of cheese and the thyme, and continue stirring until the cheese is melted. 5. In the prepared baking dish, arrange the broccoli on the bottom. Cover with half the sauce. Place the turkey pieces on top of the broccoli, and cover with the remaining sauce. Sprinkle with the remaining ¼ cup of cheese and the ground almonds. 6. Bake for 35 minutes until the sauce is bubbly and the top is browned.

Per Serving

Calories: 207 | fat: 8g | protein: 25g | carbs: 9g | sugars: 2g | fiber: 3g | sodium: 128mg

Italian Chicken Thighs

Prep time: 5 minutes | Cook time: 20 minutes | Serves 2

4 bone-in, skin-on chicken thighs
2 tablespoons unsalted butter, melted
1 teaspoon dried parsley
1 teaspoon dried basil
½ teaspoon garlic powder
¼ teaspoon onion powder
¼ teaspoon dried oregano

1. Brush chicken thighs with butter and sprinkle remaining ingredients over thighs. Place thighs into the air fryer basket. 2. Adjust the temperature to 380ºF (193ºC) and roast for 20 minutes. 3. Halfway through the cooking time, flip the thighs. 4. When fully cooked, internal temperature will be at least 165ºF (74ºC) and skin will be crispy. Serve warm.

Per Serving

Calorie: 446 | fat: 34g | protein: 33g | carbs: 2g | sugars: 0g | fiber: 0g | sodium: 163mg

Chicken with Lemon Caper Pan Sauce

Prep time: 10 minutes | Cook time: 15 minutes | Serves 4

3 tablespoons extra-virgin olive oil
4 chicken breast halves or thighs, pounded slightly to even thickness
½ teaspoon sea salt
⅛ teaspoon freshly ground

black pepper
¼ cup freshly squeezed lemon juice
¼ cup dry white wine
2 tablespoons capers, rinsed
2 tablespoons salted butter, very cold, cut into pieces

1. In a large skillet over medium-high heat, heat the olive oil until it shimmers. 2. Season the chicken with the salt and pepper. Add it to the hot oil and cook until opaque with an internal temperature of 165°F, about 5 minutes per side. Transfer the chicken to a plate and tent loosely with foil to keep warm. Keep the pan on the heat. 3. Add the lemon juice and wine to the pan, using the side of a spoon to scrape any browned bits from the bottom of the pan. Add the capers. Simmer until the liquid is reduced by half, about 3 minutes. Reduce the heat to low. 4. Whisk in the butter, one piece at a time, until incorporated. 5. Return the chicken to the pan, turning once to coat with the sauce. Serve with additional sauce spooned over the top.

Per Serving

Calorie: 367 | fat: 23g | protein: 37g | carbs: 2g | sugars: 1g | fiber: 0g | sodium: 591mg

Thanksgiving Turkey Breast

Prep time: 5 minutes | Cook time: 30 minutes | Serves 4

1½ teaspoons fine sea salt
1 teaspoon ground black pepper
1 teaspoon chopped fresh rosemary leaves
1 teaspoon chopped fresh sage
1 teaspoon chopped fresh tarragon

1 teaspoon chopped fresh thyme leaves
1 (2-pound / 907-g) turkey breast
3 tablespoons ghee or unsalted butter, melted
3 tablespoons Dijon mustard

1. Spray the air fryer with avocado oil. Preheat the air fryer to 390ºF (199ºC). 2. In a small bowl, stir together the salt, pepper, and herbs until well combined. Season the turkey breast generously on all sides with the seasoning. 3. In another small bowl, stir together the ghee and Dijon. Brush the ghee mixture on all sides of the turkey breast. 4. Place the turkey breast in the air fryer basket and air fry for 30 minutes, or until the internal temperature reaches 165ºF (74ºC). Transfer the breast to a cutting board and allow it to rest for 10 minutes before cutting it into ½-inch-thick slices. 5. Store leftovers in an airtight container in the refrigerator for up to 4 days or in the freezer for up to a month. Reheat in a preheated 350ºF (177ºC) air fryer for 4 minutes, or until warmed through.

Per Serving

Calorie: 418 | fat: 22g | protein: 51g | carbs: 1g | sugars: 0g | fiber: 1g | sodium: 603mg

Herb-Roasted Turkey and Vegetables

Prep time: 20 minutes | Cook time: 2 hours | Serves 6

2 teaspoons minced garlic
1 tablespoon chopped fresh parsley
1 teaspoon chopped fresh thyme
1 teaspoon chopped fresh rosemary
2 pounds boneless, skinless whole turkey breast
3 teaspoons extra-virgin olive oil, divided

Sea salt
Freshly ground black pepper
2 sweet potatoes, peeled and cut into 2-inch chunks
2 carrots, peeled and cut into 2-inch chunks
2 parsnips, peeled and cut into 2-inch chunks
1 sweet onion, peeled and cut into eighths

1. Preheat the oven to 350°F. 2. Line a large roasting pan with aluminum foil and set it aside. 3. In a small bowl, mix together the garlic, parsley, thyme, and rosemary. 4. Place the turkey breast in the roasting pan and rub it all over with 1 teaspoon of olive oil. 5. Rub the garlic-herb mixture all over the turkey and season lightly with salt and pepper. 6. Place the turkey in the oven and roast for 30 minutes. 7. While the turkey is roasting, toss the sweet potatoes, carrots, parsnips, onion, and the remaining 2 teaspoons of olive oil in a large bowl. 8. Remove the turkey from the oven and arrange the vegetables around it. 9. Roast until the turkey is cooked through (170°F internal temperature) and the vegetables are lightly caramelized, about 1 ½ hours.

Per Serving

Calorie: 267 | fat: 4g | protein: 35g | carbs: 25g | sugars: 8g | fiber: 5g | sodium: 379mg

Saffron-Spiced Chicken Breasts

Prep time: 10 minutes | Cook time: 10 minutes | Serves 4

Pinch saffron (3 or 4 threads)
½ cup plain nonfat yogurt
2 tablespoons water
½ onion, chopped
3 garlic cloves, minced
2 tablespoons chopped fresh cilantro

Juice of ½ lemon
½ teaspoon salt
1 pound boneless, skinless chicken breasts, cut into 2-inch strips
1 tablespoon extra-virgin olive oil

1. In a blender jar, combine the saffron, yogurt, water, onion, garlic, cilantro, lemon juice, and salt. Pulse to blend. 2. In a large mixing bowl, combine the chicken and the yogurt sauce, and stir to coat. Cover and refrigerate for at least 1 hour or up to overnight. 3. In a large skillet, heat the oil over medium heat. Add the chicken pieces, shaking off any excess marinade. Discard the marinade. Cook the chicken pieces on each side for 5 minutes, flipping once, until cooked through and golden brown.

Per Serving

Calories: 155 | fat: 5g | protein: 26g | carbs: 3g | sugars: 1g | fiber: 0g | sodium: 501mg

Smoky Chicken Leg Quarters

Prep time: 30 minutes | Cook time: 23 to 27 minutes | Serves 6

½ cup avocado oil
2 teaspoons smoked paprika
1 teaspoon sea salt
1 teaspoon garlic powder
½ teaspoon dried rosemary
½ teaspoon dried thyme
½ teaspoon freshly ground black pepper
2 pounds (907 g) bone-in, skin-on chicken leg quarters

1. In a blender or small bowl, combine the avocado oil, smoked paprika, salt, garlic powder, rosemary, thyme, and black pepper. 2. Place the chicken in a shallow dish or large zip-top bag. Pour the marinade over the chicken, making sure all the legs are coated. Cover and marinate for at least 2 hours or overnight. 3. Place the chicken in a single layer in the air fryer basket, working in batches if necessary. Set the air fryer to 400ºF (204ºC) and air fry for 15 minutes. Flip the chicken legs, then reduce the temperature to 350ºF (177ºC). Cook for 8 to 12 minutes more, until an instant-read thermometer reads 160ºF (71ºC) when inserted into the thickest piece of chicken. 4. Allow to rest for 5 to 10 minutes before serving.
Per Serving

Calorie: 347 | fat: 25g | protein: 29g | carbs: 1g | sugars: 0g | fiber: 0g | sodium: 534mg

Ginger Curry Chicken Kabobs

Prep time: 5 minutes | Cook time: 5 minutes | Serves 4

4 teaspoons fresh lemon juice
½ teaspoon cayenne pepper
¼ teaspoon freshly ground black pepper
1-inch piece of fresh ginger, peeled and minced
1 teaspoon curry powder
4 teaspoons extra-virgin olive oil
Two 8-ounce boneless, skinless chicken breasts, halved and cut into ¼-inch strips

1. In a medium bowl, combine all ingredients except the chicken. Add the chicken, and let marinate overnight in the refrigerator. 2. Thread the chicken onto metal or wooden skewers (remember to soak the wooden skewers in water before using). 3. Grill over medium heat until the chicken is no longer pink, about 15 minutes. Transfer to a platter, and serve.
Per Serving

Calorie: 180 | fat: 8g | protein: 26g | carbs: 1g | sugars: 0g | fiber: 0g | sodium: 52mg

Orange Chicken Thighs with Bell Peppers

Prep time: 15 to 20 minutes | Cook time: 7 minutes | Serves 4 to 6

6 boneless skinless chicken thighs, cut into bite-sized pieces
2 packets crystallized True Orange flavoring
½ teaspoon True Orange Orange Ginger seasoning
½ teaspoon coconut aminos
¼ teaspoon Worcestershire sauce
Olive oil or cooking spray
2 cups bell pepper strips, any color combination (I used red)
1 onion, chopped
1 tablespoon green onion, chopped fine
3 cloves garlic, minced or chopped
½ teaspoon pink salt
½ teaspoon black pepper
1 teaspoon garlic powder
1 teaspoon ground ginger
¼–½ teaspoon red pepper
flakes
2 tablespoons tomato paste
½ cup chicken bone broth or water
1 tablespoon brown sugar substitute (I use Sukrin Gold)
½ cup Seville orange spread (I use Crofter's brand)

1. Combine the chicken with the 2 packets of crystallized orange flavor, the orange ginger seasoning, the coconut aminos, and the Worcestershire sauce. Set aside. 2. Turn the Instant Pot to Sauté and add a touch of olive oil or cooking spray to the inner pot. Add in the orange ginger marinated chicken thighs. 3. Sauté until lightly browned. Add in the peppers, onion, green onion, garlic, and seasonings. Mix well. 4. Add the remaining ingredients; mix to combine. 5. Lock the lid, set the vent to sealing, set to 7 minutes. 6. Let the pressure release naturally for 2 minutes, then manually release the rest when cook time is up.
Per Serving

Calories: 120| fat: 2g | protein: 12g | carbs: 8g | sugars: 10g | fiber: 1.6g | sodium: 315mg

Fiber-Full Chicken Tostadas

Prep time: 15 minutes | Cook time: 10 minutes | Serves 4

1 tablespoon (9 g) chili powder
½ tablespoons (5 g) onion powder
1 tablespoon (9 g) paprika
1 teaspoon garlic powder
1 teaspoon ground cumin
1 teaspoon dried oregano
¼ teaspoons black pepper
¼ teaspoons sea salt
2 tablespoons (30 ml) cooking oil of choice
1 pound (454 g) boneless, skinless chicken breast, cut into 1 to 1½-inch (2.5 to 3.8-
cm) strips
8 corn tostada shells
1 (15.5-ounce [439-g]) can low-sodium pinto beans, undrained
1 cup (30 g) baby arugula leaves, coarsely chopped
1 large avocado, peeled and sliced to the desired thickness
4 tablespoons (32 g) crumbled queso fresco cheese
Jalapeño slices (optional)
Chopped onion (optional)
Diced tomatoes (optional)

1. In a small bowl, mix together the chili powder, onion powder, paprika, garlic powder, cumin, oregano, black pepper, and sea salt. Add the cooking oil and mix it with the seasonings to make a marinade. 2. Place the chicken strips in a large ziptop plastic bag, then add the marinade. Seal the bag and shake it to coat the chicken with the marinade. (If time permits, marinate the chicken for 30 to 60 minutes.) 3. Heat a large skillet over medium-high heat. Add the chicken strips and cook them for 4 to 5 minutes. Flip the chicken strips and cook them for 3 to 4 minutes, until they are cooked through and no longer pink. Set the skillet aside. 4. Line up the tostada shells on a serving tray. Place the pinto beans in a medium bowl and mash them to the desired consistency. Spread the beans on top of each tostada. Top each tostada with an equal amount of arugula, avocado slices, cheese, chicken and any desired additional toppings, then serve.
Per Serving

Calorie: 547 | fat: 27g | protein: 40g | carbs: 12g | sugars: 1g | fiber: 12g | sodium: 738mg

Asian Mushroom-Chicken Soup

Prep time: 30 minutes | Cook time: 15 minutes | Serves 6

1½ cups water
1 package (1 ounce) dried portabella or shiitake mushrooms
1 tablespoon canola oil
¼ cup thinly sliced green onions (4 medium)
2 tablespoons gingerroot, peeled, minced
3 cloves garlic, minced
1 jalapeño chile, seeded, minced
1 cup fresh snow pea pods, sliced diagonally

3 cups reduced-sodium chicken broth
1 can (8 ounces) sliced bamboo shoots, drained
2 tablespoons low-sodium soy sauce
½ teaspoon sriracha sauce
1 cup shredded cooked chicken breast
1 cup cooked brown rice
4 teaspoons lime juice
½ cup thinly sliced fresh basil leaves

1. In medium microwavable bowl, heat water uncovered on High 30 seconds or until hot. Add mushrooms; let stand 5 minutes or until tender. Drain mushrooms (reserve liquid). Slice any mushrooms that are large. Set aside. 2. In 4-quart saucepan, heat oil over medium heat. Add 2 tablespoons of the green onions, the gingerroot, garlic and chile to oil. Cook about 3 minutes, stirring occasionally, until vegetables are tender. Add snow pea pods; cook 2 minutes, stirring occasionally. Stir in mushrooms, reserved mushroom liquid and the remaining ingredients, except lime juice and basil. Heat to boiling; reduce heat. Cover and simmer 10 minutes or until hot. Stir in lime juice. 3. Divide soup evenly among 6 bowls. Top servings with basil and remaining green onions.

Per Serving

Calories: 150 | fat: 4g | protein: 11g | carbs: 16g | sugars: 3g | fiber: 3g | sodium: 490mg

Fajita-Stuffed Chicken Breast

Prep time: 15 minutes | Cook time: 25 minutes | Serves 4

2 (6-ounce / 170-g) boneless, skinless chicken breasts
¼ medium white onion, peeled and sliced
1 medium green bell pepper,

seeded and sliced
1 tablespoon coconut oil
2 teaspoons chili powder
1 teaspoon ground cumin
½ teaspoon garlic powder

1. Slice each chicken breast completely in half lengthwise into two even pieces. Using a meat tenderizer, pound out the chicken until it's about ¼-inch thickness. 2. Lay each slice of chicken out and place three slices of onion and four slices of green pepper on the end closest to you. Begin rolling the peppers and onions tightly into the chicken. Secure the roll with either toothpicks or a couple pieces of butcher's twine. 3. Drizzle coconut oil over chicken. Sprinkle each side with chili powder, cumin, and garlic powder. Place each roll into the air fryer basket. 4. Adjust the temperature to 350ºF (177ºC) and air fry for 25 minutes. 5. Serve warm.

Per Serving

Calorie: 168 | fat: 7g | protein: 25g | carbs: 3g | sugars: 1g | fiber: 1g | sodium: 320mg

Cast Iron Hot Chicken

Prep time: 10 minutes | Cook time: 40 minutes | Serves 4

2 boneless, skinless chicken breasts
Juice of 2 limes
2 garlic cloves, minced

1 medium yellow onion, chopped
1½ teaspoons cayenne pepper
1 teaspoon smoked paprika

1. Preheat the oven to 375°F. 2. In a shallow bowl, massage the chicken all over with the lime juice, garlic, onion, cayenne, and paprika. 3. In a cast iron skillet, place the chicken in one even layer. 4. Transfer the skillet to the oven and cook for 35 to 40 minutes, or until cooked through. 5. Remove the chicken from the oven, and let rest for 5 minutes. 6. Divide each breast into two portions. Serve.

Per Serving

Calorie: 286 | fat: 4g | protein: 31g | carbs: 6g | sugars: 2g | fiber: 1g | sodium: 64mg

Speedy Chicken Cacciatore

Prep time: 5 minutes | Cook time: 30 minutes | Serves 6

2 pounds boneless, skinless chicken thighs
1½ teaspoons fine sea salt
½ teaspoon freshly ground black pepper
2 tablespoons extra-virgin olive oil
3 garlic cloves, chopped
2 large red bell peppers, seeded and cut into ¼ by 2-inch strips

2 large yellow onions, sliced
½ cup dry red wine
1½ teaspoons Italian seasoning
½ teaspoon red pepper flakes (optional)
One 14½-ounce can diced tomatoes and their liquid
2 tablespoons tomato paste
Cooked brown rice or whole-grain pasta for serving

1. Season the chicken thighs on both sides with 1 teaspoon of the salt and the black pepper. 2. Select the Sauté setting on the Instant Pot and heat the oil and garlic for 2 minutes, until the garlic is bubbling but not browned. Add the bell peppers, onions, and remaining ½ teaspoon salt and sauté for 3 minutes, until the onions begin to soften. Stir in the wine, Italian seasoning, and pepper flakes (if using). Using tongs, add the chicken to the pot, turning each piece to coat it in the wine and spices and nestling them in a single layer in the liquid. Pour the tomatoes and their liquid on top of the chicken and dollop the tomato paste on top. Do not stir them in. 3. Secure the lid and set the Pressure Release to Sealing. Press the Cancel button to reset the cooking program, then select the Poultry, Pressure Cook, or Manual setting and set the cooking time for 12 minutes at high pressure. (The pot will take about 15 minutes to come up to pressure before the cooking program begins.) 4. When the cooking program ends, perform a quick pressure release by moving the Pressure Release to Venting, or let the pressure release naturally. Open the pot and, using tongs, transfer the chicken and vegetables to a serving dish. 5. Spoon some of the sauce over the chicken and serve hot, with the rice on the side.

Per Serving

Calories: 297 | fat: 11g | protein: 32g | carbs: 16g | sugars: 3g | fiber: 3g | sodium: 772mg

Chicken Paprika

Prep time: 5 minutes | Cook time: 35 minutes | Serves 8

1 tablespoon extra-virgin olive oil	1 teaspoon salt
1 large onion, minced	⅛ teaspoon freshly ground black pepper
1 medium red bell pepper, julienned	Four 8-ounce boneless, skinless chicken breasts, halved
1 cup sliced fresh mushrooms	
1–2 teaspoons smoked paprika	8 ounces plain low-fat Greek yogurt
2 tablespoons lemon juice	

1. Heat the oil in a large skillet over medium heat. Add the onion, red pepper, and mushrooms, and sauté until tender, about 3–4 minutes. 2. Add 1 cup of water, the paprika, lemon juice, salt, and pepper, blending well. Bring the mixture to a boil over high heat, and reduce the heat to medium. Add the chicken; cover, and let simmer for 25–30 minutes or until the chicken is no longer pink. 3. Reduce the heat to low, quickly stir in the Greek yogurt, mixing well, and continue to cook for 1–2 minutes. Do not boil. Serve hot.

Per Serving

Calorie: 184 | fat: 5g | protein: 29g | carbs: 4g | sugars: 3g | fiber: 1g | sodium: 209mg

Orange Chicken

Prep time: 10 minutes | Cook time: 10 minutes | Serves 4

3 tablespoons extra-virgin olive oil	Juice and zest of 1 orange
1 pound chicken breasts or thighs, cut into ¾-inch pieces	1 teaspoon cornstarch
	½ teaspoon sriracha (or to taste)
1 teaspoon peeled and grated fresh ginger	Sesame seeds (optional, for garnish)
2 garlic cloves, minced	Thinly sliced scallion (optional, for garnish)
1 tablespoon honey	

1. In a large skillet over medium-high heat, heat the olive oil until it shimmers. Add the chicken to the oil and cook, stirring occasionally, until opaque, about 5 minutes. Add the ginger and garlic and cook, stirring constantly, for 30 seconds. 2. In a small bowl, whisk together the honey, orange juice and zest, cornstarch, and sriracha. Add the sauce mixture to the chicken and cook, stirring, until the sauce thickens, about 2 minutes. 3. Serve garnished with sesame seeds and sliced scallions, if desired.

Per Serving

Calorie: 264 | fat: 15g | protein: 23g | carbs: 10g | sugars: 8g | fiber: 1g | sodium: 109mg

Chicken in Wine

Prep time: 10 minutes | Cook time: 12 minutes | Serves 6

2 pounds chicken breasts, trimmed of skin and fat	reduced-sodium cream of mushroom soup
10¾-ounce can 98% fat-free,	10¾-ounce can French onion
soup	chicken broth
1 cup dry white wine or	

1. Place the chicken into the Instant Pot. 2. Combine soups and wine. Pour over chicken. 3. Secure the lid and make sure vent is set to sealing. Cook on Manual mode for 12 minutes. 4. When cook time is up, let the pressure release naturally for 5 minutes and then release the rest manually.

Per Serving

Calories: 225 | fat: 5g | protein: 35g | carbs: 7g | sugars: 3g | fiber: 1g | sodium: 645mg

Ginger Turmeric Chicken Thighs

Prep time: 5 minutes | Cook time: 25 minutes | Serves 4

4 (4-ounce / 113-g) boneless, skin-on chicken thighs	½ teaspoon salt
	½ teaspoon garlic powder
2 tablespoons coconut oil, melted	½ teaspoon ground ginger
	¼ teaspoon ground black pepper
½ teaspoon ground turmeric	

1. Place chicken thighs in a large bowl and drizzle with coconut oil. Sprinkle with remaining ingredients and toss to coat both sides of thighs. 2. Place thighs skin side up into ungreased air fryer basket. Adjust the temperature to 400°F (204°C) and air fry for 25 minutes. After 10 minutes, turn thighs. When 5 minutes remain, flip thighs once more. Chicken will be done when skin is golden brown and the internal temperature is at least 165°F (74°C). Serve warm.

Per Serving

Calorie: 392 | fat: 31g | protein: 25g | carbs: 1g | sugars: 0g | fiber: 0g | sodium: 412mg

Jerk Chicken Thighs

Prep time: 30 minutes | Cook time: 15 to 20 minutes | Serves 6

2 teaspoons ground coriander	½ teaspoon ground cinnamon
1 teaspoon ground allspice	½ teaspoon ground nutmeg
1 teaspoon cayenne pepper	2 pounds (907 g) boneless chicken thighs, skin on
1 teaspoon ground ginger	
1 teaspoon salt	2 tablespoons olive oil
1 teaspoon dried thyme	

1. In a small bowl, combine the coriander, allspice, cayenne, ginger, salt, thyme, cinnamon, and nutmeg. Stir until thoroughly combined. 2. Place the chicken in a baking dish and use paper towels to pat dry. Thoroughly coat both sides of the chicken with the spice mixture. Cover and refrigerate for at least 2 hours, preferably overnight. 3. Preheat the air fryer to 360°F (182°C). 4. Working in batches if necessary, arrange the chicken in a single layer in the air fryer basket and lightly coat with the olive oil. Pausing halfway through the cooking time to flip the chicken, air fry for 15 to 20 minutes, until a thermometer inserted into the thickest part registers 165°F (74°C).

Per Serving

Calorie: 227 | fat: 11g | protein: 30g | carbs: 1g | sugars: 0g | fiber: 0g | sodium: 532mg

Tantalizing Jerked Chicken

Prep time: 10 minutes | Cook time: 20 minutes | Serves 4

4 (5-ounce) boneless, skinless chicken breasts
½ sweet onion, cut into chunks
2 habanero chile peppers, halved lengthwise, seeded
¼ cup freshly squeezed lime juice
2 tablespoons extra-virgin olive oil
1 tablespoon minced garlic
1 tablespoon ground allspice

2 teaspoons chopped fresh thyme
1 teaspoon freshly ground black pepper
½ teaspoon ground nutmeg
¼ teaspoon ground cinnamon
2 cups fresh greens (such as arugula or spinach)
1 cup halved cherry tomatoes

1. Place two chicken breasts in each of two large resealable plastic bags. Set them aside. 2. Place the onion, habaneros, lime juice, olive oil, garlic, allspice, thyme, black pepper, nutmeg, and cinnamon in a food processor and pulse until very well blended. 3. Pour half the marinade into each bag with the chicken breasts. Squeeze out as much air as possible, seal the bags, and place them in the refrigerator for 4 hours. 4. Preheat a barbecue to medium-high heat. 5. Let the chicken sit at room temperature for 15 minutes and then grill, turning at least once, until cooked through, about 15 minutes total. 6. Let the chicken rest for about 5 minutes before serving. Divide the greens and tomatoes among four serving plates, and top with the chicken.
Per Serving

Calorie: 268 | fat: 10g | protein: 33g | carbs: 9g | sugars: 4g | fiber: 2g | sodium: 74mg

Grain-Free Parmesan Chicken

Prep time: 5 minutes | Cook time: 20 minutes | Serves 4

1½ cups (144 g) almond flour
½ cup (50 g) grated Parmesan cheese
1 tablespoon (3 g) Italian seasoning
1 teaspoon garlic powder
½ teaspoons black pepper
2 large eggs

4 (6-ounce [170-g], ½-inch [13-mm]-thick) boneless, skinless chicken breasts
½ cup (120 ml) no-added-sugar marinara sauce
½ cup (56 g) shredded mozzarella cheese
2 tablespoons (8 g) minced fresh herbs of choice (optional)

1. Preheat the oven to 375°F (191°C). Line a large, rimmed baking sheet with parchment paper. 2. In a shallow dish, mix together the almond flour, Parmesan cheese, Italian seasoning, garlic powder, and black pepper. In another shallow dish, whisk the eggs. Dip a chicken breast into the egg wash, then gently shake off any extra egg. Dip the chicken breast into the almond flour mixture, coating it well. Place the chicken breast on the prepared baking sheet. Repeat this process with the remaining chicken breasts. 3. Bake the chicken for 15 to 20 minutes, or until the meat is no longer pink in the center. 4. Remove the chicken from the oven and flip each breast. Top each breast with 2 tablespoons (30 ml) of marinara sauce and 2 tablespoons (14 g) of mozzarella cheese. 5. Increase the oven temperature to broil and place the chicken back in the oven. Broil it until the cheese is melted and just starting to brown. Carefully remove the chicken from the oven, top it with the herbs (if using), and let it rest for about 10 minutes before serving.
Per Serving

Calorie: 572 | fat: 32g | protein: 60g | carbs: 13g | sugars: 4g | fiber:5g | sodium: 560mg

Herbed Whole Turkey Breast

Prep time: 10 minutes | Cook time:30 minutes | Serves 12

3 tablespoons extra-virgin olive oil
1½ tablespoons herbes de Provence or poultry seasoning
2 teaspoons minced garlic
1 teaspoon lemon zest (from 1 small lemon)

1 tablespoon kosher salt
1½ teaspoons freshly ground black pepper
1 (6-pound) bone-in, skin-on whole turkey breast, rinsed and patted dry

1. In a small bowl, whisk together the olive oil, herbes de Provence, garlic, lemon zest, salt, and pepper. 2. Rub the outside of the turkey and under the skin with the olive oil mixture. 3. Pour 1 cup of water into the electric pressure cooker and insert a wire rack or trivet. 4. Place the turkey on the rack, skin-side up. 5. Close and lock the lid of the pressure cooker. Set the valve to sealing. 6. Cook on high pressure for 30 minutes. 7. When the cooking is complete, hit Cancel. Allow the pressure to release naturally for 20 minutes, then quick release any remaining pressure. 8. Once the pin drops, unlock and remove the lid. 9. Carefully transfer the turkey to a cutting board. Remove the skin, slice, and serve.
Per Serving

Calorie: 389 | fat: 19g | protein: 50g | carbs: 1g | sugars: 0g | fiber: 0g | sodium: 582mg

Chapter 6 Fish and Seafood

Spicy Citrus Sole   61

Asian Salmon in a Packet   61

Roasted Salmon with Honey-Mustard Sauce   61

Baked Oysters   61

Quick Shrimp Skewers   62

Teriyaki Salmon   62

Shrimp with Tomatoes and Feta   62

Spicy Shrimp Fajitas   62

Broiled Sole with Mustard Sauce   62

Mediterranean Salmon with Whole-Wheat Couscous   63

Mediterranean-Style Cod   63

Roasted Tilapia and Vegetables   63

Savory Shrimp   63

Grilled Rosemary Swordfish   64

Almond Pesto Salmon   64

Crab-Stuffed Avocado Boats   64

Tuna Steak   64

Roasted Halibut with Red Peppers, Green Beans, and Onions   64

Chili Tilapia   64

Shrimp Burgers with Fruity Salsa and Salad   65

Salmon en Papillote   65

Lemon Pepper Tilapia with Broccoli and Carrots   65

Blackened Pollock   66

Creamy Cod with Asparagus   66

Crispy Fish Sticks   66

Friday Night Fish Fry   66

Air Fryer Fish Fry   66

Tilapia with Pecans   67

Scallops and Asparagus Skillet   67

Halibut with Lime and Cilantro   67

Salmon Florentine   67

Greek Scampi   67

Ginger-Glazed Salmon and Broccoli   68

Seafood Stew   68

Calypso Shrimp with Black Bean Salsa   68

Citrus-Glazed Salmon   68

Grilled Salmon with Dill Sauce   69

Baked Garlic Scampi   69

Catfish with Corn and Pepper Relish   69

Lobster Fricassee   69

Tomato Tuna Melts   69

Spicy Citrus Sole

Prep time: 10 minutes | Cook time: 10 minutes | Serves 4

1 teaspoon chili powder
1 teaspoon garlic powder
½ teaspoon lime zest
½ teaspoon lemon zest
¼ teaspoon freshly ground black pepper
¼ teaspoon smoked paprika

Pinch sea salt
4 (6-ounce) sole fillets, patted dry
1 tablespoon extra-virgin olive oil
2 teaspoons freshly squeezed lime juice

1. Preheat the oven to 450°F. 2. Line a baking sheet with aluminum foil and set it aside. 3. In a small bowl, stir together the chili powder, garlic powder, lime zest, lemon zest, pepper, paprika, and salt until well mixed. 4. Pat the fish fillets dry with paper towels, place them on the baking sheet, and rub them lightly all over with the spice mixture. 5. Drizzle the olive oil and lime juice on the top of the fish. 6. Bake until the fish flakes when pressed lightly with a fork, about 8 minutes. Serve immediately.

Per Serving

Calories: 155 | fat: 7g | protein: 21g | carbs: 1g | sugars: 0g | fiber: 1g | sodium: 524mg

Asian Salmon in a Packet

Prep time: 10 minutes | Cook time: 20 minutes | Serves 2

For the sauce
1 tablespoon extra-virgin olive oil, divided
1 teaspoon grated fresh ginger
1 garlic clove, minced
2 tablespoons low-sodium soy sauce
2 teaspoons dark sesame oil
For the salmon packets
1 teaspoon extra-virgin olive oil, divided
1 cup cooked brown rice,

divided
2 cups coarsely chopped bok choy, divided
1 small red bell pepper, sliced, divided
½ cup sliced shiitake mushrooms, divided
2 (6-ounce) salmon steaks, rinsed
2 scallions, chopped, divided

To make the sauce In a small bowl, whisk together the olive oil, ginger, garlic, soy sauce, and sesame oil. Set aside. To make the salmon packets 1. Preheat the oven to 450°F. 2. Fold 2 (12-by-24-inch) aluminum foil sheets in half widthwise into 2 (12-by-12-inch) squares. 3. Brush ½ teaspoon of the olive oil in the center of each foil square. 4. Spread ½ cup of the rice in the center of each square. 5. Over the rice in each packet, layer 1 cup of bok choy, half of the red bell pepper slices, ¼ cup of mushrooms, 1 salmon steak, and half of the scallions. 6. Pour half of the sauce over each. 7. Fold and seal the foil into airtight packets. Place the packets in a baking dish and into the preheated oven. Bake for 20 minutes. 8. Carefully avoiding the steam that will be released, open a packet and check that the fish is cooked. It should be opaque and flake easily. To test for doneness, poke the tines of a fork into the thickest portion of the fish at a 45-degree angle. Gently twist the fork and pull up some of the fish. If the fish resists flaking, return it to the oven for another 2 minutes then test again. Fish cooks very quickly, so be careful not to overcook it. 9. Transfer the contents of the packets to serving plates or bowls. 10. Enjoy!

Per Serving Calories: 491 | fat: 22g | protein: 41g | carbs: 31g | sugars: 4g | fiber: 5g | sodium: 595mg

Roasted Salmon with Honey-Mustard Sauce

Prep time: 5 minutes | Cook time: 20 minutes | Serves 4

Nonstick cooking spray
2 tablespoons whole-grain mustard
1 tablespoon honey
2 garlic cloves, minced

¼ teaspoon salt
¼ teaspoon freshly ground black pepper
1 pound salmon fillet

1. Preheat the oven to 425°F. Spray a baking sheet with nonstick cooking spray. 2. In a small bowl, whisk together the mustard, honey, garlic, salt, and pepper. 3. Place the salmon fillet on the prepared baking sheet, skin-side down. Spoon the sauce onto the salmon and spread evenly. 4. Roast for 15 to 20 minutes, depending on the thickness of the fillet, until the flesh flakes easily.

Per Serving

Calories: 186 | fat: 7g | protein: 23g | carbs: 6g | sugars: 4g | fiber: 0g | sodium: 312mg

Baked Oysters

Prep time: 30 minutes | Cook time: 15 minutes | Serves 2

2 cups coarse salt, for holding the oysters
1 dozen fresh oysters, scrubbed
1 tablespoon butter
½ cup finely chopped artichoke hearts
¼ cup finely chopped scallions, both white and green

parts
¼ cup finely chopped red bell pepper
1 garlic clove, minced
1 tablespoon finely chopped fresh parsley
Zest and juice of ½ lemon
Pinch salt
Freshly ground black pepper

1. Pour the coarse salt into an 8-by-8-inch baking dish and spread to evenly fill the bottom of the dish. 2. Prepare a clean surface to shuck the oysters. Using a shucking knife, insert the blade at the joint of the shell, where it hinges open and shut. Firmly apply pressure to pop the blade in, and work the knife around the shell to open. Discard the empty half of the shell. Use the knife to gently loosen the oyster, and remove any shell particles. Set the oysters in their shells on the salt, being careful not to spill the juices. 3. Preheat the oven to 425°F. 4. In a large skillet, melt the butter over medium heat. Add the artichoke hearts, scallions, and bell pepper, and cook for 5 to 7 minutes. Add the garlic and cook an additional minute. Remove from the heat and mix in the parsley, lemon zest and juice, and season with salt and pepper. 5. Divide the vegetable mixture evenly among the oysters and bake for 10 to 12 minutes until the vegetables are lightly browned.

Per Serving

Calories: 134 | fat: 7g | protein: 6g | carbs: 11g | sugars: 7g | fiber: 2g | sodium: 281mg

Chapter 6 Fish and Seafood | 61

Quick Shrimp Skewers

Prep time: 10 minutes | Cook time: 5 minutes | Serves 5

4 pounds (1.8 kg) shrimp, peeled
1 tablespoon dried rosemary

1 tablespoon avocado oil
1 teaspoon apple cider vinegar

1. Mix the shrimps with dried rosemary, avocado oil, and apple cider vinegar. 2. Then sting the shrimps into skewers and put in the air fryer. 3. Cook the shrimps at 400ºF (204ºC) for 5 minutes.

Per Serving

Calories: 336 | fat: 5g | protein: 73g | carbs: 0g | sugars: 0g | fiber: 0g | sodium: 432mg

Teriyaki Salmon

Prep time: 30 minutes | Cook time: 12 minutes | Serves 4

4 (6-ounce / 170-g) salmon fillets
½ cup soy sauce
¼ cup packed light brown sugar
2 teaspoons rice vinegar
1 teaspoon minced garlic

¼ teaspoon ground ginger
2 teaspoons olive oil
½ teaspoon salt
¼ teaspoon freshly ground black pepper
Oil, for spraying

1. Place the salmon in a small pan, skin-side up. 2. In a small bowl, whisk together the soy sauce, brown sugar, rice vinegar, garlic, ginger, olive oil, salt, and black pepper. 3. Pour the mixture over the salmon and marinate for about 30 minutes. 4. Line the air fryer basket with parchment and spray lightly with oil. Place the salmon in the prepared basket, skin-side down. You may need to work in batches, depending on the size of your air fryer. 5. Air fry at 400ºF (204ºC) for 6 minutes, brush the salmon with more marinade, and cook for another 6 minutes, or until the internal temperature reaches 145ºF (63ºC). Serve immediately.

Per Serving

Calories: 319 | fat: 14g | protein: 37g | carbs: 8g | sugars: 6g | fiber: 1g | sodium: 762mg

Shrimp with Tomatoes and Feta

Prep time: 10 minutes | Cook time: 30 minutes | Serves 4

3 tomatoes, coarsely chopped
½ cup chopped sun-dried tomatoes
2 teaspoons minced garlic
2 teaspoons extra-virgin olive oil
1 teaspoon chopped fresh oregano

Freshly ground black pepper
1½ pounds (16–20 count) shrimp, peeled, deveined, tails removed
4 teaspoons freshly squeezed lemon juice
½ cup low-sodium feta cheese, crumbled

1. Heat the oven to 450°F. 2. In a medium bowl, toss the tomatoes, sun-dried tomatoes, garlic, oil, and oregano until well combined. 3. Season the mixture lightly with pepper. 4. Transfer the tomato mixture to a 9-by-13-inch glass baking dish. 5. Bake until softened, about 15 minutes. 6. Stir the shrimp and lemon juice into the hot tomato mixture and top evenly with the feta. 7. Bake until the shrimp are cooked through, about 15 minutes more.

Per Serving

Calories: 252 | fat: 8g | protein: 39g | carbs: 9g | sugars: 6g | fiber: 2g | sodium: 396mg

Spicy Shrimp Fajitas

Prep time: 30 minutes | Cook time: 20 minutes | Makes 6 fajitas

Marinade
1 tablespoon lime juice
1 tablespoon olive or canola oil
¼ teaspoon salt
1 teaspoon chili powder
1 teaspoon ground cumin
2 cloves garlic, crushed
Pinch ground red pepper (cayenne)
Fajitas

2 pounds uncooked deveined peeled medium shrimp, thawed if frozen, tail shells removed
2 medium red bell peppers, cut into strips (2 cups)
1 medium red onion, sliced (2 cups)
Olive oil cooking spray
6 flour tortillas (8 inch)
¾ cup refrigerated guacamole (from 14-ounce package)

1 Heat gas or charcoal grill. In 1-gallon resealable food-storage plastic bag, mix marinade ingredients. Add shrimp; seal bag and toss to coat. Set aside while grilling vegetables, turning bag once. 2 In medium bowl, place bell peppers and onion; spray with cooking spray. Place vegetables in grill basket (grill "wok"). Wrap tortillas in foil; set aside. 3 Place basket on grill rack over medium heat. Cover grill; cook 10 minutes, turning vegetables once. 4 Drain shrimp; discard marinade. Add shrimp to grill basket. Cover grill; cook 5 to 7 minutes longer, turning shrimp and vegetables once, until shrimp are pink. Place wrapped tortillas on grill. Cook 2 minutes, turning once, until warm. 5 On each tortilla, place shrimp, vegetables and guacamole; fold tortilla over filling.

Per ServingCalories: 310 | fat: 10g | protein:27g | carbs: 29g | sugars: 4g | fiber: 2g | sodium: 770mg

Broiled Sole with Mustard Sauce

Prep time: 5 minutes | Cook time: 20 minutes | Serves 6

Nonstick cooking spray
1½ pound fresh sole filets
3 tablespoons low-fat mayonnaise
2 tablespoons Dijon mustard

2 tablespoons chopped parsley
⅛ teaspoon freshly ground black pepper
1 large lemon, cut into wedges

1. Preheat broiler. Coat a baking sheet with nonstick cooking spray. Arrange the filets so they don't overlap. 2. In a small bowl, combine the mayonnaise, mustard, parsley, and pepper, and mix thoroughly. Spread the mixture evenly over the filets. Broil 3–4 inches from the heat for 4 minutes until the fish flakes easily with a fork. 3. Arrange the filets on a serving platter, garnish with lemon wedges, and serve.

Per ServingCalories: 104 | fat: 4g | protein: 14g | carbs: 3g | sugars: 1g | fiber: 1g | sodium: 402mg

Mediterranean Salmon with Whole-Wheat Couscous

Prep time: 5 minutes | Cook time: 30 minutes | Serves 4

Couscous
1 cup whole-wheat couscous
1 cup water
1 tablespoon extra-virgin olive oil
1 teaspoon dried basil
¼ teaspoon fine sea salt
1 pint cherry or grape tomatoes, halved
8 ounces zucchini, halved lengthwise, then sliced crosswise ¼ inch thick

Salmon
1 pound skinless salmon fillet
2 teaspoons extra-virgin olive oil
1 tablespoon fresh lemon juice
1 garlic clove, minced
¼ teaspoon dried oregano
¼ teaspoon fine sea salt
¼ teaspoon freshly ground black pepper
1 tablespoon capers, drained
Lemon wedges for serving

1. Pour 1 cup water into the Instant Pot. Have ready two-tier stackable stainless-steel containers. 2. To make the couscous: In one of the containers, stir together the couscous, water, oil, basil, and salt. Sprinkle the tomatoes and zucchini over the top. 3. To make the salmon: Place the salmon fillet in the second container. In a small bowl, whisk together the oil, lemon juice, garlic, oregano, salt, pepper, and capers. Spoon the oil mixture over the top of the salmon. 4. Place the container with the couscous and vegetables on the bottom and the salmon container on top. Cover the top container with its lid and then latch the containers together. Grasping the handle, lower the containers into the Instant Pot. 5. Secure the lid and set the Pressure Release to Sealing. Select the Pressure Cook or Manual setting and set the cooking time for 20 minutes at high pressure. (The pot will take about 10 minutes to come up to pressure before the cooking program begins.) 6. When the cooking program ends, let the pressure release naturally for 5 minutes, then move the Pressure Release to Venting to release any remaining steam. Open the pot and, wearing heat-resistant mitts, lift out the stacked containers. Unlatch, unstack, and open the containers, taking care not to get burned by the steam. 7. Using a fork, fluff the couscous and mix in the vegetables. Spoon the couscous onto plates, then use a spatula to cut the salmon into four pieces and place a piece on top of each couscous serving. Serve right away, with lemon wedges on the side.
Per Serving Calories: 427 | fat: 18g | protein: 28g | carbs: 36g | sugars: 2g | fiber: 6g | sodium: 404mg

Mediterranean-Style Cod

Prep time: 5 minutes | Cook time: 12 minutes | Serves 4

4 (6-ounce / 170-g) cod fillets
3 tablespoons fresh lemon juice
1 tablespoon olive oil

¼ teaspoon salt
6 cherry tomatoes, halved
¼ cup pitted and sliced kalamata olives

1. Place cod into an ungreased round nonstick baking dish. Pour lemon juice into dish and drizzle cod with olive oil. Sprinkle with salt. Place tomatoes and olives around baking dish in between fillets. 2. Place dish into air fryer basket. Adjust the temperature to 350°F (177°C) and bake for 12 minutes, carefully turning cod halfway through cooking. Fillets will be lightly browned, easily flake, and have an internal temperature of at least 145°F (63°C) when done. Serve warm.
Per Serving Calories: 186 | fat: 5g | protein: 31g | carbs: 2g | sugars: 1g | fiber: 1g | sodium: 300mg

Roasted Tilapia and Vegetables

Prep time: 15 minutes | Cook time: 20 minutes | Serves 4

½ pound fresh asparagus spears, trimmed, halved
2 small zucchini, halved lengthwise, cut into ½-inch pieces
1 red bell pepper, cut into ½-inch strips
1 large onion, cut into ½-inch wedges

1 tablespoon olive oil
2 teaspoons Montreal steak seasoning
4 tilapia fillets (about 1½ pounds)
2 teaspoons butter or margarine, melted
½ teaspoon paprika

1. Heat oven to 450°F. In large bowl, toss asparagus, zucchini, bell pepper, onion and oil. Sprinkle with 1 teaspoon of the steak seasoning; toss to coat. Spread vegetables in ungreased 15x10x1-inch pan. Place on lower oven rack; roast 5 minutes. 2. Meanwhile, spray 13x9-inch (3-quart) glass baking dish with cooking spray. Pat tilapia fillets dry with paper towels. Brush with butter; sprinkle with remaining 1 teaspoon steak seasoning and the paprika. Place in baking dish. 3. Place baking dish on middle oven rack. Roast fish and vegetables 17 to 18 minutes longer or until fish flakes easily with fork and vegetables are tender.
Per Serving

Calories: 250 | fat: 8g | protein: 35g | carbs: 10g | sugars: 5g | fiber: 3g | sodium: 160mg

Savory Shrimp

Prep time: 5 minutes | Cook time: 8 to 10 minutes | Serves 4

1 pound (454 g) fresh large shrimp, peeled and deveined
1 tablespoon avocado oil
2 teaspoons minced garlic, divided
½ teaspoon red pepper flakes

Sea salt and freshly ground black pepper, to taste
2 tablespoons unsalted butter, melted
2 tablespoons chopped fresh parsley

1. Place the shrimp in a large bowl and toss with the avocado oil, 1 teaspoon of minced garlic, and red pepper flakes. Season with salt and pepper. 2. Set the air fryer to 350°F (177°C). Arrange the shrimp in a single layer in the air fryer basket, working in batches if necessary. Cook for 6 minutes. Flip the shrimp and cook for 2 to 4 minutes more, until the internal temperature of the shrimp reaches 120°F (49°C). (The time it takes to cook will depend on the size of the shrimp.) 3. While the shrimp are cooking, melt the butter in a small saucepan over medium heat and stir in the remaining 1 teaspoon of garlic. 4. Transfer the cooked shrimp to a large bowl, add the garlic butter, and toss well. Top with the parsley and serve warm.
Per Serving

Calories: 182 | fat: 10g | protein: 23g | carbs: 1g | sugars: 0g | fiber: 0g | sodium: 127mg

Grilled Rosemary Swordfish

Prep time: 5 minutes | Cook time: 15 minutes | Serves 4

2 scallions, thinly sliced
2 tablespoons extra-virgin olive oil
2 tablespoons white wine vinegar

1 teaspoon fresh rosemary, finely chopped
4 swordfish steaks (1 pound total)

1. In a small bowl, combine the scallions, olive oil, vinegar, and rosemary. Pour over the swordfish steaks. Let the steaks marinate for 30 minutes. 2. Remove the steaks from the marinade, and grill for 5–7 minutes per side, brushing with marinade. Transfer to a serving platter, and serve.

Per Serving

Calories: 225 | fat: 14g | protein: 22g | carbs: 0g | sugars: 0g | fiber: 0g | sodium: 92mg

Almond Pesto Salmon

Prep time: 5 minutes | Cook time: 12 minutes | Serves 2

¼ cup pesto
¼ cup sliced almonds, roughly chopped
2 (1½-inch-thick) salmon

fillets (about 4 ounces / 113 g each)
2 tablespoons unsalted butter, melted

1. In a small bowl, mix pesto and almonds. Set aside. 2. Place fillets into a round baking dish. 3. Brush each fillet with butter and place half of the pesto mixture on the top of each fillet. Place dish into the air fryer basket. 4. Adjust the temperature to 390ºF (199ºC) and set the timer for 12 minutes. 5. Salmon will easily flake when fully cooked and reach an internal temperature of at least 145ºF (63ºC). Serve warm.

Per Serving

Calories: 478 | fat: 39g | protein: 29g | carbs: 4g | sugars: 1g | fiber: 2g | sodium: 366mg

Crab-Stuffed Avocado Boats

Prep time: 5 minutes | Cook time: 7 minutes | Serves 4

2 medium avocados, halved and pitted
8 ounces (227 g) cooked crab meat

¼ teaspoon Old Bay seasoning
2 tablespoons peeled and diced yellow onion
2 tablespoons mayonnaise

1. Scoop out avocado flesh in each avocado half, leaving ½ inch around edges to form a shell. Chop scooped-out avocado. 2. In a medium bowl, combine crab meat, Old Bay seasoning, onion, mayonnaise, and chopped avocado. Place ¼ mixture into each avocado shell. 3. Place avocado boats into ungreased air fryer basket. Adjust the temperature to 350ºF (177ºC) and air fry for 7 minutes. Avocado will be browned on the top and mixture will be bubbling when done. Serve warm.

Per Serving

Calories: 226 | fat: 17g | protein: 12g | carbs: 10g | sugars: 1g | fiber: 7g | sodium: 239mg

Tuna Steak

Prep time: 10 minutes | Cook time: 12 minutes | Serves 4

1 pound (454 g) tuna steaks, boneless and cubed
1 tablespoon mustard

1 tablespoon avocado oil
1 tablespoon apple cider vinegar

1. Mix avocado oil with mustard and apple cider vinegar. 2. Then brush tuna steaks with mustard mixture and put in the air fryer basket. 3. Cook the fish at 360ºF (182ºC) for 6 minutes per side.

Per Serving

Calories: 197 | fat: 9g | protein: 27g | carbs: 0g | sugars: 0g | fiber: 0g | sodium: 87mg

Roasted Halibut with Red Peppers, Green Beans, and Onions

Prep time: 10 minutes | Cook time: 15 minutes | Serves 4

1 pound green beans, trimmed
2 red bell peppers, seeded and cut into strips
1 onion, sliced
Zest and juice of 2 lemons
3 garlic cloves, minced
2 tablespoons extra-virgin

olive oil
1 teaspoon dried dill
1 teaspoon dried oregano
4 (4-ounce) halibut fillets
½ teaspoon salt
¼ teaspoon freshly ground black pepper

1. Preheat the oven to 400°F. Line a baking sheet with parchment paper. 2. In a large bowl, toss the green beans, bell peppers, onion, lemon zest and juice, garlic, olive oil, dill, and oregano. 3. Use a slotted spoon to transfer the vegetables to the prepared baking sheet in a single layer, leaving the juice behind in the bowl. 4. Gently place the halibut fillets in the bowl, and coat in the juice. Transfer the fillets to the baking sheet, nestled between the vegetables, and drizzle them with any juice left in the bowl. Sprinkle the vegetables and halibut with the salt and pepper. 5. Bake for 15 to 20 minutes until the vegetables are just tender and the fish flakes apart easily.

Per Serving

Calories: 234 | fat: 9g | protein: 24g | carbs: 16g | sugars: 8g | fiber: 5g | sodium: 349mg

Chili Tilapia

Prep time: 5 minutes | Cook time: 20 minutes | Serves 4

4 tilapia fillets, boneless
1 teaspoon chili flakes
1 teaspoon dried oregano

1 tablespoon avocado oil
1 teaspoon mustard

1. Rub the tilapia fillets with chili flakes, dried oregano, avocado oil, and mustard and put in the air fryer. 2. Cook it for 10 minutes per side at 360ºF (182ºC).

Per Serving

Calories: 146 | fat: 6g | protein: 23g | carbs: 1g | sugars: 0g | fiber: 0g | sodium: 94mg

Shrimp Burgers with Fruity Salsa and Salad

Prep time: 15 minutes | Cook time: 10 minutes | Serves 4

For the salsa
1 cup diced mango
1 avocado, diced
1 scallion, both white and green parts, finely chopped
1 tablespoon chopped fresh cilantro
Juice of 1 lime
¼ teaspoon freshly ground black pepper
For the burgers
1 pound shrimp, peeled and deveined

1 large egg
½ red bell pepper, seeded and coarsely chopped
¼ cup chopped scallions, both white and green parts
2 tablespoons fresh chopped cilantro
2 garlic cloves
¼ teaspoon freshly ground black pepper
1 tablespoon extra-virgin olive oil
4 cups mixed salad greens

To make the salsa 1. In a small bowl, toss the mango, avocado, scallion, and cilantro. Sprinkle with the lime juice and pepper. Mix gently to combine and set aside. To make the burgers 2. In the bowl of a food processor, add half the shrimp and process until coarsely puréed. Add the egg, bell pepper, scallions, cilantro, and garlic, and process until uniformly chopped. Transfer to a large mixing bowl. 3. Using a sharp knife, chop the remaining half pound of shrimp into small pieces. Add to the puréed mixture and stir well to combine. Add the pepper and stir well. Form the mixture into 4 patties of equal size. Arrange on a plate, cover, and refrigerate for 30 minutes. 4. In a large skillet, heat the olive oil over medium heat. Cook the burgers for 3 minutes on each side until browned and cooked through. 5. On each of 4 plates, arrange 1 cup of salad greens, and top with a scoop of salsa and a shrimp burger.

Per Serving

Calories: 229 | fat: 11g | protein: 19g | carbs: 14g | sugars: 7g | fiber: 4g | sodium: 200mg

Salmon en Papillote

Prep time: 15 minutes | Cook time: 15 minutes | Serves 2

For the roasted vegetables
½ pound fresh green beans, trimmed
½ onion, cut into ¼-inch-thick slices
1 tablespoon extra-virgin olive oil
1 teaspoon capers (optional)
For the salmon
2 teaspoons extra-virgin olive oil, divided
2 medium parsnips, cut into

¼-inch-thick rounds, divided
2 (4-ounce) salmon fillets
2 garlic cloves, thinly sliced, divided
1 lemon, divided (½ cut into slices, the other ½ cut into 2 wedges)
1 tablespoon chopped fresh thyme, divided
Kosher salt
Freshly ground black pepper

To make the roasted vegetables 1. Preheat the oven to 400°F. Line a baking sheet with parchment paper. 2. In a medium bowl, toss the green beans, onion, extra-virgin olive oil, and capers (if using) until well coated. 3. Spread the vegetables on half of the baking sheet and set aside until the salmon is ready to bake.

To make the salmon 4. Cut two pieces of parchment paper, fold them in half, and cut each into a heart shape (about 10 to 12 inches in circumference). Lightly brush the parchment with ½ teaspoon of extra-virgin olive oil. 5. Open one of the hearts and place half the parsnips on the right half in the center, fanning them out. Place one piece of salmon on the fanned parsnips. Add half the garlic, half the lemon slices, half the thyme, ½ teaspoon of extra-virgin olive oil, and a pinch each of kosher salt and pepper. 6. Seal the packet by folding the left half of the heart over the right side. Fold along the edge of the heart and create a seal. Repeat with the other piece of parchment. 7. Place the packets on the empty side of the baking sheet and bake until the salmon is cooked through, 10 to 15 minutes. Allow the fish to rest a few minutes before serving with the roasted green beans and remaining lemon wedges. 8. Store any leftovers in an airtight container in the refrigerator for 1 to 2 days.

Per Serving

Calories: 389 | fat: 17g | protein: 28g | carbs: 35g | sugars: 11g | fiber: 10g | sodium: 261mg

Lemon Pepper Tilapia with Broccoli and Carrots

Prep time: 0 minutes | Cook time: 15 minutes | Serves 4

1 pound tilapia fillets
1 teaspoon lemon pepper seasoning
¼ teaspoon fine sea salt
2 tablespoons extra-virgin olive oil
2 garlic cloves, minced
1 small yellow onion, sliced

½ cup low-sodium vegetable broth
2 tablespoons fresh lemon juice
1 pound broccoli crowns, cut into bite-size florets
8 ounces carrots, cut into ¼-inch thick rounds

1. Sprinkle the tilapia fillets all over with the lemon pepper seasoning and salt. 2. Select the Sauté setting on the Instant Pot and heat the oil and garlic for 2 minutes, until the garlic is bubbling but not browned. Add the onion and sauté for about 3 minutes more, until it begins to soften. 3. Pour in the broth and lemon juice, then use a wooden spoon to nudge any browned bits from the bottom of the pot. Using tongs, add the fish fillets to the pot in a single layer; it's fine if they overlap slightly. Place the broccoli and carrots on top. 4. Secure the lid and set the Pressure Release to Sealing. Press the Cancel button to reset the cooking program, then select the Pressure Cook or Manual setting and set the cooking time for 1 minute at low pressure. (The pot will take about 10 minutes to come up to pressure before the cooking program begins.) 5. When the cooking program ends, let the pressure release naturally for 10 minutes (don't open the pot before the 10 minutes are up, even if the float valve has gone down), then move the Pressure Release to Venting to release any remaining steam. Open the pot. Use a fish spatula to transfer the vegetables and fillets to plates. Serve right away.

Per Serving

Calories: 243 | fat: 9g | protein: 28g | carbs: 15g | sugars: 4g | fiber: 5g | sodium: 348mg

Chapter 6 Fish and Seafood | 65

Blackened Pollock

Prep time: 15 minutes | Cook time: 10 minutes | Serves 2

8 ounces pollock (or other white fish) fillet, skinned and halved
3 teaspoons extra-virgin olive oil, divided
1 teaspoon blackening seasoning, or Cajun seasoning, divided

¼ cup thinly sliced onion
4 cups baby spinach, divided
½ small grapefruit, peeled and segmented
2 tablespoons shaved fennel
2 tablespoons pepitas
½ small avocado, peeled, pitted, and sliced, divided

1. Brush both sides of each pollock half with 1½ teaspoons of olive oil. 2. Rub each half all over with ½ teaspoon of blackening seasoning. 3. In a large heavy skillet set over high heat, cook the pollock and onions for 2 to 3 minutes, until blackened. Turn the fillets. Cook for 2 to 3 minutes more, or until blackened and the fish flakes easily with a fork. 4. Put 2 cups of arugula on each serving plate. Top each with 1 pollock half. 5. Top each serving with half of the grapefruit, fennel, pepitas, and avocado.
Per Serving

Calories: 302 | fat: 19g | protein: 20g | carbs: 16g | sugars: 5g | fiber: 8g | sodium: 436mg

Creamy Cod with Asparagus

Prep time: 5 minutes | Cook time: 15 minutes | Serves 4

½ cup uncooked brown rice or quinoa
4 (4-ounce) cod fillets
¼ teaspoon salt
¼ teaspoon freshly ground black pepper

½ teaspoon garlic powder, divided
24 asparagus spears
Avocado oil cooking spray
1 cup half-and-half

1. Cook the rice according to the package instructions. 2. Meanwhile, season both sides of the cod fillets with the salt, pepper, and ¼ teaspoon of garlic powder. 3. Cut the bottom 1½ inches from the asparagus. 4. Heat a large pan over medium-low heat. When hot, coat the cooking surface with cooking spray, and arrange the cod and asparagus in a single layer. 5. Cover and cook for 8 minutes. 6. Add the half-and-half and the remaining ¼ teaspoon of garlic powder and stir. Increase the heat to high and simmer for 2 minutes. 7. Divide the rice, cod, and asparagus into four equal portions.
Per Serving

Calories: 219 | fat: 2g | protein: 24g | carbs: 24g | sugars: 4g | fiber: 1g | sodium: 267mg

Crispy Fish Sticks

Prep time: 15 minutes | Cook time: 10 minutes | Serves 4

1 ounce (28 g) pork rinds, finely ground
¼ cup blanched finely ground almond flour
½ teaspoon Old Bay seasoning

1 tablespoon coconut oil
1 large egg
1 pound (454 g) cod fillet, cut into ¾-inch strips

1. Place ground pork rinds, almond flour, Old Bay seasoning, and coconut oil into a large bowl and mix together. In a medium bowl, whisk egg. 2. Dip each fish stick into the egg and then gently press into the flour mixture, coating as fully and evenly as possible. Place fish sticks into the air fryer basket. 3. Adjust the temperature to 400°F (204°C) and air fry for 10 minutes or until golden. 4. Serve immediately.
Per Serving

Calories: 223 | fat: 14g | protein: 21g | carbs: 2g | sugars: 0g | fiber: 1g | sodium: 390mg

Friday Night Fish Fry

Prep time: 10 minutes | Cook time: 10 minutes | Serves 4

1 large egg
½ cup powdered Parmesan cheese (about 1½ ounces / 43 g)
1 teaspoon smoked paprika
¼ teaspoon celery salt
¼ teaspoon ground black

pepper
4 (4-ounce / 113-g) cod fillets
Chopped fresh oregano or parsley, for garnish (optional)
Lemon slices, for serving (optional)

1. Spray the air fryer basket with avocado oil. Preheat the air fryer to 400°F (204°C). 2. Crack the egg in a shallow bowl and beat it lightly with a fork. Combine the Parmesan cheese, paprika, celery salt, and pepper in a separate shallow bowl. 3. One at a time, dip the fillets into the egg, then dredge them in the Parmesan mixture. Using your hands, press the Parmesan onto the fillets to form a nice crust. As you finish, place the fish in the air fryer basket. 4. Air fry the fish in the air fryer for 10 minutes, or until it is cooked through and flakes easily with a fork. Garnish with fresh oregano or parsley and serve with lemon slices, if desired. 5. Store leftovers in an airtight container in the refrigerator for up to 3 days. Reheat in a preheated 400°F (204°C) air fryer for 5 minutes, or until warmed through.
Per Serving

Calories: 165 | fat: 6g | protein: 25g | carbs: 2g | sugars: 0g | fiber: 0g | sodium: 392mg

Air Fryer Fish Fry

Prep time: 5 minutes | Cook time: 15 minutes | Serves 4

2 cups low-fat buttermilk
½ teaspoon garlic powder
½ teaspoon onion powder
4 (4-ounce) flounder fillets

½ cup plain yellow cornmeal
½ cup chickpea flour
¼ teaspoon cayenne pepper
Freshly ground black pepper

1. In a large bowl, combine the buttermilk, garlic powder, and onion powder. 2. Add the flounder, turning until well coated, and set aside to marinate for 20 minutes. 3. In a shallow bowl, stir the cornmeal, chickpea flour, cayenne, and pepper together. 4. Dredge the fillets in the meal mixture, turning until well coated. Place in the basket of an air fryer. 5. Set the air fryer to 380°F, close, and cook for 12 minutes.
Per Serving

Calories: 266 | fat: 7g | protein: 27g | carbs: 24g | sugars: 8g | fiber: 2g | sodium: 569mg

Tilapia with Pecans

Prep time: 20 minutes | Cook time: 16 minutes | Serves 5

2 tablespoons ground flaxseeds
1 teaspoon paprika
Sea salt and white pepper, to taste
1 teaspoon garlic paste
2 tablespoons extra-virgin olive oil
½ cup pecans, ground
5 tilapia fillets, sliced into halves

1. Combine the ground flaxseeds, paprika, salt, white pepper, garlic paste, olive oil, and ground pecans in a Ziploc bag. Add the fish fillets and shake to coat well. 2. Spritz the air fryer basket with cooking spray. Cook in the preheated air fryer at 400°F (204°C) for 10 minutes; turn them over and cook for 6 minutes more. Work in batches. 3. Serve with lemon wedges, if desired. Enjoy!

Per Serving

Calories: 252 | fat: 17g | protein: 25g | carbs: 3g | sugars: 1g | fiber: 2g | sodium: 65mg

Scallops and Asparagus Skillet

Prep time: 10 minutes | Cook time: 15 minutes | Serves 4

3 teaspoons extra-virgin olive oil, divided
1 pound asparagus, trimmed and cut into 2-inch segments
1 tablespoon butter
1 pound sea scallops
¼ cup dry white wine
Juice of 1 lemon
2 garlic cloves, minced
¼ teaspoon freshly ground black pepper

1. In a large skillet, heat 1½ teaspoons of oil over medium heat. 2. Add the asparagus and sauté for 5 to 6 minutes until just tender, stirring regularly. Remove from the skillet and cover with aluminum foil to keep warm. 3. Add the remaining 1½ teaspoons of oil and the butter to the skillet. When the butter is melted and sizzling, place the scallops in a single layer in the skillet. Cook for about 3 minutes on one side until nicely browned. Use tongs to gently loosen and flip the scallops, and cook on the other side for another 3 minutes until browned and cooked through. Remove and cover with foil to keep warm. 4. In the same skillet, combine the wine, lemon juice, garlic, and pepper. Bring to a simmer for 1 to 2 minutes, stirring to mix in any browned pieces left in the pan. 5. Return the asparagus and the cooked scallops to the skillet to coat with the sauce. Serve warm.

Per Serving

Calories: 252 | fat: 7g | protein: 26g | carbs: 15g | sugars: 3g | fiber: 2g | sodium: 493mg

Halibut with Lime and Cilantro

Prep time: 30 minutes | Cook time: 10 to 20 minutes | Serves 2

2 tablespoons lime juice
1 tablespoon chopped fresh cilantro
1 teaspoon olive or canola oil
1 clove garlic, finely chopped
2 halibut or salmon steaks (about ¾ pounds)
Freshly ground pepper to taste
½ cup chunky-style salsa

1. In shallow glass or plastic dish or in resealable food-storage plastic bag, mix lime juice, cilantro, oil and garlic. Add halibut, turning several times to coat with marinade. Cover; refrigerate 15 minutes, turning once. 2. Heat gas or charcoal grill. Remove halibut from marinade; discard marinade. 3. Place halibut on grill over medium heat. Cover grill; cook 10 to 20 minutes, turning once, until halibut flakes easily with fork. Sprinkle with pepper. Serve with salsa.

Per Serving

Calories: 190 | fat: 4.5g | protein: 32g | carbs: 6g | sugars: 2g | fiber: 0g | sodium: 600mg

Salmon Florentine

Prep time: 10 minutes | Cook time: 30 minutes | Serves 4

1 teaspoon extra-virgin olive oil
½ sweet onion, finely chopped
1 teaspoon minced garlic
3 cups baby spinach
1 cup kale, tough stems
removed, torn into 3-inch pieces
Sea salt
Freshly ground black pepper
4 (5-ounce) salmon fillets
Lemon wedges, for serving

1. Preheat the oven to 350°F. 2. Place a large skillet over medium-high heat and add the oil. 3. Sauté the onion and garlic until softened and translucent, about 3 minutes. 4. Add the spinach and kale and sauté until the greens wilt, about 5 minutes. 5. Remove the skillet from the heat and season the greens with salt and pepper. 6. Place the salmon fillets so they are nestled in the greens and partially covered by them. Bake the salmon until it is opaque, about 20 minutes. 7. Serve immediately with a squeeze of fresh lemon.

Per Serving

Calories: 211 | fat: 8g | protein: 30g | carbs: 5g | sugars: 2g | fiber: 1g | sodium: 129mg

Greek Scampi

Prep time: 10 minutes | Cook time: 5 minutes | Serves 2

2 garlic cloves, minced
2 tablespoons extra-virgin olive oil
½ pound shrimp, peeled, deveined, and thoroughly rinsed
1 cup diced tomatoes
½ cup nonfat ricotta cheese
6 Kalamata olives
Juice of ½ lemon
2 teaspoons chopped fresh dill, or ¾ teaspoon dried
Dash salt
Dash freshly ground black pepper
Lemon wedges, for garnish

1. In a large skillet set over medium heat, sauté the garlic in the olive oil for 30 seconds. 2. Add the shrimp. Cook for 1 minute. 3. Add the tomatoes, ricotta cheese, olives, lemon juice, and dill. Reduce the heat to low. Simmer for 5 to 10 minutes, stirring so the shrimp cook on both sides. When the shrimp are pink and the tomatoes and ricotta have made a sauce, the dish is ready. 4. Sprinkle with salt and pepper. 5. Serve immediately, garnished with lemon wedges.

Per Serving

Calories: 345 | fat: 21g | protein: 31g | carbs: 11g | sugars: 3g | fiber: 2g | sodium: 406mg

Ginger-Glazed Salmon and Broccoli

Prep time: 10 minutes | Cook time: 15 minutes | Serves 4

Nonstick cooking spray
1 tablespoon low-sodium tamari or gluten-free soy sauce
Juice of 1 lemon
1 tablespoon honey
1 (1-inch) piece fresh ginger, grated
1 garlic clove, minced
1 pound salmon fillet
¼ teaspoon salt, divided
⅛ teaspoon freshly ground black pepper
2 broccoli heads, cut into florets
1 tablespoon extra-virgin olive oil

1. Preheat the oven to 400°F. Spray a baking sheet with nonstick cooking spray. 2. In a small bowl, mix the tamari, lemon juice, honey, ginger, and garlic. Set aside. 3. Place the salmon skin-side down on the prepared baking sheet. Season with ⅛ teaspoon of salt and the pepper. 4. In a large mixing bowl, toss the broccoli and olive oil. Season with the remaining ⅛ teaspoon of salt. Arrange in a single layer on the baking sheet next to the salmon. Bake for 15 to 20 minutes until the salmon flakes easily with a fork and the broccoli is fork-tender. 5. In a small pan over medium heat, bring the tamari-ginger mixture to a simmer and cook for 1 to 2 minutes until it just begins to thicken. 6. Drizzle the sauce over the salmon and serve.

Per Serving

Calories: 238 | fat: 11g | protein: 25g | carbs: 11g | sugars: 6g | fiber: 2g | sodium: 334mg

Seafood Stew

Prep time: 20 minutes | Cook time: 30 minutes | Serves 6

1 tablespoon extra-virgin olive oil
1 sweet onion, chopped
2 teaspoons minced garlic
3 celery stalks, chopped
2 carrots, peeled and chopped
1 (28-ounce) can sodium-free diced tomatoes, undrained
3 cups low-sodium chicken broth
½ cup clam juice
¼ cup dry white wine
2 teaspoons chopped fresh basil
2 teaspoons chopped fresh oregano
2 (4-ounce) haddock fillets, cut into 1-inch chunks
1 pound mussels, scrubbed, debearded
8 ounces (16–20 count) shrimp, peeled, deveined, quartered
Sea salt
Freshly ground black pepper
2 tablespoons chopped fresh parsley

1. Place a large saucepan over medium-high heat and add the olive oil. 2. Sauté the onion and garlic until softened and translucent, about 3 minutes. 3. Stir in the celery and carrots and sauté for 4 minutes. 4. Stir in the tomatoes, chicken broth, clam juice, white wine, basil, and oregano. 5. Bring the sauce to a boil, then reduce the heat to low. Simmer for 15 minutes. 6. Add the fish and mussels, cover, and cook until the mussels open, about 5 minutes. 7. Discard any unopened mussels. Add the shrimp to the pan and cook until the shrimp are opaque, about 2 minutes. 8. Season with salt and pepper. Serve garnished with the chopped parsley.

Per Serving

Calories: 230 | fat: 6g | protein: 27g | carbs: 18g | sugars: 8g | fiber: 4g | sodium: 490mg

Calypso Shrimp with Black Bean Salsa

Prep time: 25 minutes | Cook time: 5 minutes | Serves 4

Shrimp
½ teaspoon grated lime peel
1 tablespoon lime juice
1 tablespoon canola oil
1 teaspoon finely chopped gingerroot
1 clove garlic, finely chopped
1 pound uncooked deveined peeled large shrimp, thawed if frozen
Salsa
1 can (15 ounces) black beans, drained, rinsed
1 medium mango, peeled, pitted and chopped (1 cup)
1 small red bell pepper, chopped (½ cup)
2 medium green onions, sliced (2 tablespoons)
1 tablespoon chopped fresh cilantro
½ teaspoon grated lime peel
1 to 2 tablespoons lime juice
1 tablespoon red wine vinegar
¼ teaspoon ground red pepper (cayenne)

1. In medium glass or plastic bowl, mix lime peel, lime juice, oil, gingerroot and garlic. Stir in shrimp; let stand 15 minutes. 2. Meanwhile, in medium bowl, mix salsa ingredients. 3. In 10-inch skillet, cook shrimp over medium-high heat about 5 minutes, turning once, until pink. Serve with salsa.

Per Serving

Calories: 300| fat: 5g | protein: 26g | carbs: 37g | sugars: 7g | fiber: 12g | sodium: 190mg

Citrus-Glazed Salmon

Prep time: 10 minutes | Cook time: 13 to 17 minutes | Serves 4

2 medium limes
1 small orange
⅓ cup agave syrup
1 teaspoon salt
1 teaspoon pepper
4 cloves garlic, finely chopped
1¼ pounds salmon fillet, cut
into 4 pieces
2 tablespoons sliced green onions
1 lime slice, cut into 4 wedges
1 orange slice, cut into 4 wedges
Hot cooked orzo pasta or rice, if desired

1. Heat oven to 400°F. Line 15x10x1-inch pan with cooking parchment paper or foil. In small bowl, grate lime peel from limes. Squeeze enough lime juice to equal 2 tablespoons; add to peel in bowl. Grate orange peel from oranges into bowl. Squeeze enough orange juice to equal 2 tablespoons; add to peel mixture. Stir in agave syrup, salt, pepper and garlic. In small cup, measure ¼ cup citrus mixture for salmon (reserve remaining citrus mixture). 2. Place salmon fillets in pan, skin side down. Using ¼ cup citrus mixture, brush tops and sides of salmon. Bake 13 to 17 minutes or until fish flakes easily with fork. Lift salmon pieces from skin with metal spatula onto serving plate. Sprinkle with green onions. Top each fish fillet with lime and orange wedges. Serve each fillet with 3 tablespoons reserved sauce and rice.

Per Serving

Calories: 320 | fat: 8g | protein: 31g | carbs: 30g | sugars: 23g | fiber: 3g | sodium: 680mg

Grilled Salmon with Dill Sauce

Prep time: 10 minutes | Cook time: 15 minutes | Serves 8

1 cup plain fat-free Greek yogurt
2 teaspoons minced fresh dill
¼ cup chopped scallions or onion
1 teaspoon capers
2 teaspoons minced fresh

parsley
1 teaspoon minced fresh chives
Nonstick cooking spray
2 pounds salmon steaks
1 tablespoon extra-virgin olive oil

1. In a small bowl, combine the yogurt, dill, scallions or onion, capers, parsley, and chives; set aside. 2. Spray the racks of your grill with nonstick cooking spray. 3. Brush the salmon steaks with olive oil, and grill them over medium-hot coals for 4 minutes per side, or just until the salmon flakes with a fork. 4. Transfer the salmon to a platter, and serve with the dill sauce on the side.

Per Serving

Calories: 181 | fat: 7g | protein: 25g | carbs: 3g | sugars: 2g | fiber: 0g | sodium: 116mg

Baked Garlic Scampi

Prep time: 5 minutes | Cook time: 10 minutes | Serves 4

1 tablespoon extra-virgin olive oil
¼ teaspoon salt
7 garlic cloves, crushed
2 tablespoons chopped fresh

parsley, divided
1 pound large shrimp, shelled (with tails left on) and deveined
Juice and zest of 1 lemon
2 cups baby arugula

1. Preheat the oven to 350 degrees. Grease a 13-x-9-x-2-inch baking pan with the olive oil. Add the salt, garlic, and 1 tablespoon of the parsley in a medium bowl; mix well, and set aside. 2. Arrange the shrimp in a single layer in the baking pan, and bake for 3 minutes, uncovered. Turn the shrimp, and sprinkle with the lemon peel, lemon juice, and the remaining 1 tablespoon of parsley. Continue to bake 1–2 minutes more until the shrimp are bright pink and tender. 3. Remove the shrimp from the oven. Place the arugula on a serving platter, and top with the shrimp. Spoon the garlic mixture over the shrimp and arugula, and serve.

Per Serving

Calories: 140 | fat: 4g | protein: 23g | carbs: 3g | sugars: 1g | fiber: 0g | sodium: 285mg

Catfish with Corn and Pepper Relish

Prep time: 10 minutes | Cook time: 10 minutes | Serves 4

3 tablespoons extra-virgin olive oil, divided
4 (5-ounce) catfish fillets
¼ teaspoon salt
¼ teaspoon freshly ground black pepper

1 (15-ounce) can low-sodium black beans, drained and rinsed
1 cup frozen corn
1 medium red bell pepper, diced

1 tablespoon apple cider vinegar

3 tablespoons chopped scallions

1. Use 1½ tablespoons of oil to coat both sides of the catfish fillets, then season the fillets with the salt and pepper. 2. Heat a small saucepan over medium-high heat. Put the remaining 1½ tablespoons of oil, beans, corn, bell pepper, and vinegar in the pan and stir. Cover and cook for 5 minutes. 3. Place the catfish fillets on top of the relish mixture and cover. Cook for 5 to 7 minutes. 4. Serve each catfish fillet with one-quarter of the relish and top with the scallions.

Per Serving

Calories: 379 | fat: 15g | protein: 32g | carbs: 31g | sugars: 2g | fiber: 10g | sodium: 366mg

Lobster Fricassee

Prep time: 5 minutes | Cook time: 20 minutes | Serves 4

2 cups shelled lobster meat
1 tablespoon extra-virgin olive oil
¾ pound mushrooms, sliced
1 small onion, minced
½ cup fat-free milk
¼ cup flour

¼ teaspoon paprika
¼ teaspoon salt
⅛ teaspoon freshly ground black pepper
2 cups cooked whole-wheat pasta
¼ cup finely chopped parsley

1. Cut the lobster meat into bite-size pieces. In a saucepan, heat the oil; add the mushrooms and onion, and sauté for 5–6 minutes. 2. In a small bowl, whisk the milk and flour, whisking quickly to eliminate any lumps. Pour the milk mixture into the mushroom mixture; mix thoroughly, and continue cooking for 3–5 minutes. 3. Add the lobster, paprika, salt, and pepper; continue cooking for 5–10 minutes until the lobster is heated through. 4. Spread the pasta onto a serving platter, spoon the lobster and sauce over the top, and garnish with parsley to serve.

Per Serving

Calories: 248 | fat: 5g | protein: 22g | carbs: 31g | sugars: 5g | fiber: 5g | sodium: 523mg

Tomato Tuna Melts

Prep time: 5 minutes | Cook time: 5 minutes | Serves 2

1 (5-ounce) can chunk light tuna packed in water, drained
2 tablespoons plain nonfat Greek yogurt
2 teaspoons freshly squeezed lemon juice
2 tablespoons finely chopped celery

1 tablespoon finely chopped red onion
Pinch cayenne pepper
1 large tomato, cut into ¾-inch-thick rounds
½ cup shredded cheddar cheese

1. Preheat the broiler to high. 2. In a medium bowl, combine the tuna, yogurt, lemon juice, celery, red onion, and cayenne pepper. Stir well. 3. Arrange the tomato slices on a baking sheet. Top each with some tuna salad and cheddar cheese. 4. Broil for 3 to 4 minutes until the cheese is melted and bubbly. Serve.

Per Serving

Calories: 243 | fat: 10g | protein: 30g | carbs: 7g | sugars: 2g | fiber: 1g | sodium: 444mg

Chapter 7 Salads

Italian Potato Salad 71

Lentil Salad 71

Garden-Fresh Greek Salad 71

Pomegranate "Tabbouleh" with
Cauliflower 71

Herbed Spring Peas 71

Tortilla-Bean Salad 72

Salmon Niçoise Salad 72

Cheeseburger Wedge Salad 72

Nutty Deconstructed Salad 72

Rainbow Quinoa Salad 73

Roasted Carrot and Quinoa with Goat
Cheese 73

Chicken Tender and Brussels Sprout
Cobb Salad 73

Curried Chicken Salad 73

Roasted Asparagus–Berry Salad 74

Mediterranean Chef Salad 74

Make-Ahead Apple, Carrot, and Cabbage
Slaw 74

Crab and Rice Salad 74

Greek Rice Salad 74

Strawberry-Spinach Salad 75

Quinoa, Beet, and Greens Salad 75

Broccoli Slaw Crab Salad 75

otisserie Chicken and Avocado Salad 75

Shaved Brussels Sprouts and Kale with
Poppy Seed Dressing 75

Chickpea Salad 76

Cabbage Slaw Salad 76

Apple-Bulgur Salad 76

Romaine Lettuce Salad with Cranberry,
Feta, and Beans 76

Sweet Beet Grain Bowl 76

Sunflower-Tuna-Cauliflower Salad 77

Power Salad 77

Grilled Romaine with White Beans 77

Greek Island Potato Salad 77

Chinese Chicken Salad 77

Grilled Hearts of Romaine with Buttermilk
Dressing 78

Three Bean and Basil Salad 78

Chickpea "Tuna" Salad 78

Lentil-Apple Salad 78

First-of-the-Season Tomato, Peach, and
Strawberry Salad 78

Edamame and Walnut Salad 79

Zucchini, Carrot, and Fennel Salad 79

Italian Potato Salad

Prep time: 10 minutes | Cook time: 25 minutes | Serves 8

12 new red potatoes, 3–4 ounces each, washed and skins left on
3 celery stalks, chopped
1 red bell pepper, minced
¼ cup chopped scallions
2 tablespoons olive oil
1 tablespoon balsamic vinegar
½ tablespoon red vinegar
1 teaspoon chopped fresh parsley
⅛ teaspoon freshly ground black pepper

1. Boil the potatoes for 20 minutes in a large pot of boiling water. Drain, and let cool for 30 minutes. 2. Cut the potatoes into large chunks, and toss the potatoes with the celery, bell pepper, and scallions. 3. In a medium bowl, combine the olive oil, balsamic vinegar, red vinegar, parsley, and pepper; pour the dressing over the potato salad. Serve at room temperature.

Per Serving

Calorie: 128 | fat: 4g | protein: 3g | carbs: 22g | sugars: 3g | fiber: 3g | sodium: 30mg

Lentil Salad

Prep time: 10 minutes | Cook time: 45 minutes | Serves 8

1 pound dried lentils, washed (rinse with cold water in a colander)
3 cups water
2 tablespoons extra-virgin olive oil
2 teaspoons cumin
1 teaspoon minced fresh oregano
3 tablespoons fresh lemon
juice
¼ teaspoon freshly ground black pepper
2 large green bell peppers, cored, seeded, and diced
2 large red bell peppers, cored, seeded, and diced
3 stalks celery, diced
1 red onion, minced

1. In a large saucepan over high heat, bring lentils and water to a boil. Reduce the heat to low, cover, and simmer for 35–45 minutes. Drain, and set aside. 2. In a large bowl, mix together the oil, cumin, oregano, lemon juice, and pepper until well blended. Add the lentils and the prepared vegetables. Cover, and chill in the refrigerator before serving.

Per Serving

Calorie: 261 | fat: 4g | protein: 15g | carbs: 43g | sugars: 5g | fiber: 8g | sodium: 15mg

Garden-Fresh Greek Salad

Prep time: 20 minutes | Cook time: 0 minutes | Serves 6

Dressing
3 tablespoons fresh lemon juice
1 tablespoon chopped fresh or 1 teaspoon dried oregano leaves
½ teaspoon salt
½ teaspoon sugar
½ teaspoon Dijon mustard
¼ teaspoon pepper
1 clove garlic, finely chopped
Salad
1 bag (10 ounces) ready-to-eat romaine lettuce
¾ cup chopped seeded peeled cucumber
½ cup sliced red onion
¼ cup sliced kalamata olives
2 medium tomatoes, seeded,
chopped (1½ cups)
¼ cup reduced-fat feta cheese

1. In small bowl, beat all dressing ingredients with whisk. 2. In large bowl, toss all salad ingredients except cheese. Stir in dressing until salad is well coated. Sprinkle with cheese.

Per Serving

Calorie: 45 | fat: 1.5g | protein: 3g | carbs: 6g | sugars: 3g | fiber: 2g | sodium: 340mg

Pomegranate "Tabbouleh" with Cauliflower

Prep time: 20 minutes | Cook time: 5 minutes | Serves 4 to 6

⅓ cup extra-virgin olive oil, divided
4 cups grated cauliflower (about 1 medium head)
Juice of 1 lemon
¼ red onion, minced
4 large tomatoes, diced
3 large bunches flat-leaf parsley, chopped
1 large bunch mint, chopped
½ cup pomegranate arils
Kosher salt
Freshly ground black pepper

1. In a large skillet, heat 2 tablespoons of extra-virgin olive oil. When it's hot, add the cauliflower and sauté for 3 to 5 minutes or until it starts to crisp. Remove the skillet from the heat and allow the cauliflower to cool while you prep the remaining ingredients. 2. In a large bowl, combine the remaining extra-virgin olive oil with the lemon juice and red onion. Mix well, then mix in the tomatoes, parsley, mint, and pomegranate arils. 3. After the cauliflower cools, 5 to 7 minutes, add it to the bowl with the other ingredients. Season with salt and pepper to taste and serve. 4. Store any leftovers in an airtight container in the refrigerator for 3 to 5 days.

Per Serving

Calorie: 205 | fat: 15g | protein: 4g | carbs: 17g | sugars: 9g | fiber: 5g | sodium: 50mg

Herbed Spring Peas

Prep time: 10 minutes | Cook time: 15 minutes | Serves 6

1 tablespoon unsalted non-hydrogenated plant-based butter
½ Vidalia onion, thinly sliced
1 cup store-bought low-sodium
vegetable broth
3 cups fresh shelled peas
1 tablespoon minced fresh tarragon

1. In a skillet, melt the butter over medium heat. 2. Add the onion and sauté for 2 to 3 minutes, or until the onion is translucent. 3. Add the broth, and reduce the heat to low. 4. Add the peas and tarragon, cover, and cook for 7 to 10 minutes, or until the peas soften. 5. Serve.

Per Serving

Calorie: 43 | fat: 2g | protein: 2g | carbs: 6g | sugars: 3g | fiber: 2g | sodium: 159mg

Tortilla-Bean Salad

Prep time: 15 minutes | Cook time: 0 minutes | Serves 4

½ cup bottled French-style salad dressing
1 (15-ounce) can black beans, rinsed and drained
1 large tomato, diced
1 large green bell pepper, seeded and cut into large chunks
1 small onion, chopped

1 avocado, peeled, pitted, and cubed
1 (8-ounce) package shredded taco cheese
4 cups mixed salad greens
1 cup tricolor tortilla strips, divided
4 tablespoons salsa, divided (optional)

1. Pour the salad dressing into a large bowl. Add the beans, tomato, bell pepper, onion, avocado, and cheese. Mix to coat the ingredients with dressing. 2. Add the salad greens and mix again to coat. 3. Portion into 4 servings and top each with ¼ cup of tortilla strips. 4. Garnish each serving with 1 tablespoon of salsa, if desired.

Per Serving

Calorie: 504 | fat: 28g | protein: 23g | carbs: 44g | sugars: 10g | fiber: 15g | sodium: 546mg

Salmon Niçoise Salad

Prep time: 10 minutes | Cook time: 30 minutes | Serves 1

Salad
4 ounces (113 g) fresh salmon fillets
Cooking oil spray, as needed
1 teaspoon olive oil
Sea salt, as needed
Black pepper, as needed
2 cups (60 g) arugula
⅛ cup (17 g) assorted olives
½ cup (60 g) coarsely chopped cucumber
1 large hard-boiled egg
½ cup (65 g) quartered baby potatoes

2 teaspoons (2 g) dried rosemary
2½ ounces (71 g) fresh green beans
Dressing
1 tablespoon (15 g) tahini
½ tablespoons (8 g) Dijon mustard
1 tablespoon (15 ml) fresh lemon juice
3 tablespoons (45 ml) water
½ teaspoons dried dill
Sea salt, as needed
Black pepper, as needed

1. Preheat the oven to 400°F (204°C). Line a large baking sheet with parchment paper. 2. Bring a large pot of water to a boil over high heat. 3. To make the salad, heat a medium skillet over medium-high heat. Spray the salmon with the cooking oil spray and drizzle the oil on top. Place it in the skillet and cook for 2 to 3 minutes on each side (depending how thick the fillet is), until the outside is an opaque pink color and just barely starts to brown. Season the salmon with the salt and black pepper. 4. On a serving plate, arrange a bed of arugula. On the arugula, arrange the olives, cucumber, egg, and salmon. Set the plate aside. 5. Place the potatoes in a medium bowl. Add the rosemary and toss to coat the potatoes. Transfer them to the prepared baking sheet and bake them for 20 to 25 minutes, or until the potatoes are brown and crispy on the outside. 6. While the potatoes are roasting, prepare a large bowl of ice water. Add the green beans to the boiling water and cook them for 2 minutes. Quickly transfer the green beans to the bowl of ice water. Once they have cooled, add the green beans to the salad. 7. To make the dressing, mix together the tahini, mustard, lemon juice, water, dill, sea salt, and black pepper in a medium jar. 8. Add the potatoes to the salad, toss the salad with the dressing, and serve.

Per Serving

Calorie: 471 | fat: 23g | protein: 37g | carbs: 31g | sugars: 6g | fiber: 7g | sodium: 555mg

Cheeseburger Wedge Salad

Prep time: 15 minutes | Cook time: 10 minutes | Serves 4

Salad
1 pound (454 g) lean ground beef
2 medium heads romaine lettuce, rinsed, dried, and sliced in half lengthwise
½ cup (60 g) shredded Cheddar cheese
½ cup (80 g) coarsely chopped tomatoes
⅓ cup (50 g) finely chopped red onion

1 small dill pickle, finely chopped (optional)
Dressing
2 ounces (57 g) no-salt-added tomato paste
2 tablespoons (30 ml) apple cider vinegar
2 tablespoons (30 ml) water
1 tablespoon (15 ml) honey
¼ teaspoons sea salt
½ teaspoons onion powder
¼ teaspoons garlic powder

1. To make the salad, heat a large skillet over medium-high heat. Once the skillet is hot, add the beef and cook it for 9 to 10 minutes, until it is brown and cooked though. 2. Meanwhile, place a ½ head of romaine lettuce on each of four plates. Divide the beef evenly on top of each of the romaine halves. Then top each with the Cheddar cheese, tomatoes, onion, and pickle (if using). 3. To make the dressing, combine the tomato paste, vinegar, water, honey, sea salt, onion powder, and garlic powder in a small mason jar, secure the lid on top, and shake the jar thoroughly until everything is combined. Drizzle the dressing evenly over each salad and serve.

Per Serving

Calorie: 320 | fat: 14g | protein: 32g | carbs: 19g | sugars: 11g | fiber: 8g | sodium: 341mg

Nutty Deconstructed Salad

Prep time: 10 minutes | Cook time: 0 minutes | Serves 1

6 ounces (170 g) grilled or baked chicken, sliced or cubed to the desired size
½ cup (75 g) red seedless grapes
¼ cup (32 g) crumbled feta

cheese
¼ cup (30 g) raw walnuts
2 tablespoons (10 g) raw pumpkin seeds
1 small apple, thinly sliced

1. In a salad bowl, combine the chicken, grapes, feta cheese, walnuts, pumpkin seeds, and apple. Toss to combine the ingredients and serve.

Per Serving

Calorie: 613 | fat: 33g | protein: 42g | carbs: 42g | sugars: 30g | fiber: 6g | sodium: 501mg

Rainbow Quinoa Salad

Prep time: 10 minutes | Cook time: 0 minutes | Serves 3

Dressing
3½ tablespoons orange juice
1 tablespoon apple cider vinegar
1 tablespoon pure maple syrup
1½ teaspoons yellow mustard
Couple pinches of cloves
Rounded ½ teaspoon sea salt
Freshly ground black pepper to taste
Salad
2 cups cooked quinoa, cooled

½ cup corn kernels
½ cup diced apple tossed in ½ teaspoon lemon juice
¼ cup diced red pepper
¼ cup sliced green onions or chives
1 can (15 ounces) black beans, rinsed and drained
Sea salt to taste
Freshly ground black pepper to taste

1. To make the dressing: In a large bowl, whisk together the orange juice, vinegar, syrup, mustard, cloves, salt, and pepper. 2. To make the salad: Add the quinoa, corn, apple, red pepper, green onion or chives, and black beans, and stir to combine well. Season with the salt and black pepper to taste. Serve, or store in an airtight container in the fridge.

Per Serving

Calorie: 355 | fat: 4g | protein: 15g | carbs: 68g | sugars: 12g | fiber: 15g | sodium: 955mg

Roasted Carrot and Quinoa with Goat Cheese

Prep time: 10 minutes | Cook time: 20 minutes | Serves 4

4 large carrots, cut into ⅛-inch-thick rounds
4 tablespoons oil (olive, safflower, or grapeseed), divided
2 teaspoons paprika
1 teaspoon turmeric

2 teaspoons ground cumin
2 cups water
1 cup quinoa, rinsed
½ cup shelled pistachios, toasted
4 ounces goat cheese
12 ounces salad greens

1. Preheat the oven to 400°F. Line a baking sheet with parchment paper. 2. In a large bowl, toss together the carrots, 2 tablespoons of oil, the paprika, turmeric, and cumin until the carrots are well coated. Spread them evenly on the prepared baking sheet and roast until tender, 15 to 17 minutes. 3. In a medium saucepan, combine the water and quinoa over high heat. Bring to a boil, reduce the heat to low and simmer until tender, about 15 minutes. 4. Transfer the roasted carrots to a large bowl and add the cooked quinoa, remaining 2 tablespoons of oil, the pistachios, and goat cheese and toss to combine. 5. Evenly divide the greens among four plates and top with the carrot mixture. Serve. 6. Store any leftovers in an airtight container in the refrigerator for up to 2 days.

Per Serving

Calorie: 544 | fat: 33g | protein: 21g | carbs: 43g | sugars: 6g | fiber: 9g | sodium: 202mg

Chicken Tender and Brussels Sprout Cobb Salad

Prep time: 10 minutes | Cook time: 30 minutes | Serves 4

For the salad
8 (2-ounce) chicken tenders
Avocado oil cooking spray
2 (9-ounce) packages shaved Brussels sprouts
2 hardboiled eggs, chopped
½ cup unsweetened dried

cranberries
For the dressing
3 tablespoons honey mustard
3 tablespoons extra-virgin olive oil
½ tablespoon freshly squeezed lemon juice

To make the salad 1. Preheat the oven to 425°F. 2. Lightly coat the chicken tenders with cooking spray, then place them on a baking sheet and bake for 15 to 18 minutes. 3. When the chicken is done, cut the chicken tenders into even pieces. Divide the Brussels sprouts into four equal portions. Top each portion with one-quarter of the chopped eggs, dried cranberries, and 2 sliced chicken tenders. 5. Drizzle an equal portion of dressing over each serving. To make the dressing 6. In a small bowl, whisk together the mustard, olive oil, and lemon juice.

Per Serving

Calorie: 340 | fat: 17g | protein: 35g | carbs: 14g | sugars: 4g | fiber: 6g | sodium: 312mg

Curried Chicken Salad

Prep time: 15 minutes | Cook time: 40 minutes | Serves 2

4 ounces chicken breast, rinsed and drained
1 small apple, peeled, cored, and finely chopped
2 tablespoons slivered almonds
1 tablespoon dried cranberries
2 tablespoons chia seeds
¼ cup plain nonfat Greek

yogurt
1 tablespoon curry powder
1½ teaspoons Dijon mustard
⅛ teaspoon salt
¼ teaspoon freshly ground black pepper
4 cups chopped romaine lettuce, divided

1. Preheat the oven to 400°F. 2. To a small baking dish, add the chicken. Place the dish in the preheated oven. Bake for 30 to 40 minutes, or until the chicken is completely opaque and registers 165°F on an instant-read thermometer. Remove from the oven. Chop into cubes. Set aside. 3. In a medium bowl, mix together the chicken, apple, almonds, cranberries, and chia seeds. 4. Add the yogurt, curry powder, mustard, salt, and pepper. Toss to coat. 5. On 2 plates, arrange 2 cups of lettuce on each. 6. Top each with one-half of the curried chicken salad. 7. Serve immediately.

Per Serving

Calorie: 240 | fat: 9g | protein: 19g | carbs: 25g | sugars: 14g | fiber: 8g | sodium: 258mg

Roasted Asparagus–Berry Salad

Prep time: 10 minutes | Cook time: 18 minutes | Serves 4

1 pound fresh asparagus spears
Cooking spray
2 tablespoons chopped pecans
1 cup sliced fresh strawberries

4 cups mixed salad greens
¼ cup fat-free balsamic vinaigrette dressing
Cracked pepper, if desired

1. Heat oven to 400°F. Line 15x10x1-inch pan with foil; spray with cooking spray. Break off tough ends of asparagus as far down as stalks snap easily. Cut into 1-inch pieces. 2. Place asparagus in single layer in pan; spray with cooking spray. Place pecans in another shallow pan. 3. Bake pecans 5 to 6 minutes or until golden brown, stirring occasionally. Bake asparagus 10 to 12 minutes or until crisp-tender. Cool pecans and asparagus 8 to 10 minutes or until room temperature. 4. In medium bowl, mix asparagus, pecans, strawberries, greens and dressing. Sprinkle with pepper.

Per Serving

Calorie: 90 | fat: 3g | protein: 4g | carbs: 11g | sugars: 6g | fiber: 4g | sodium: 180mg

Mediterranean Chef Salad

Prep time: 20 minutes | Cook time: 0 minutes | Serves 4

½ cup extra-virgin olive oil
½ cup red wine vinegar
2 tablespoons grated Parmesan cheese
1 teaspoon dried Italian herb blend
1 (15-ounce) can chickpeas, rinsed and drained
1 medium cucumber, peeled

and diced
½ cup diced roasted red peppers
½ cup pitted and sliced kalamata olives
½ cup crumbled feta cheese
4 cups spinach, romaine, and arugula salad mix, divided

1. In large bowl, whisk together the olive oil, red wine vinegar, Parmesan cheese, and Italian herbs. 2. Add the chickpeas, cucumber, red peppers, olives, and feta cheese and mix until everything is coated well. 3. Divide the greens into 4 bowls and top each with 1 cup of the salad mix.

Per Serving

Calorie: 318 | fat: 22g | protein: 10g | carbs: 20g | sugars: 5g | fiber: 7g | sodium: 510mg

Make-Ahead Apple, Carrot, and Cabbage Slaw

Prep time: 10 minutes | Cook time: 0 minutes | Serves 6

4 cups shredded cabbage (green or purple, or a mixture)
2 cups shredded carrots
¾ cup sliced scallions
¾ cup unsweetened apple juice
⅔ cup cider vinegar
1½ teaspoons paprika

1 teaspoon mustard seeds
½ teaspoon garlic powder
½ teaspoon celery seeds
⅛ teaspoon freshly ground black pepper
1 tablespoon dry mustard

1. In a large bowl, combine the cabbage, carrots, and scallions. 2. In a blender, combine the remaining ingredients. Pour over the cabbage mixture, and toss to coat. Refrigerate overnight, and serve chilled.

Per Serving

Calorie: 57 | fat: 1g | protein: 2g | carbs: 12g | sugars: 7g | fiber: 3g | sodium: 68mg

Crab and Rice Salad

Prep time: 10 minutes | Cook time: 50 minutes | Serves 4

1 cup uncooked brown rice
5 ounces cooked fresh crabmeat, flaked
1 large tomato, diced
One 1.8-ounce can sliced water chestnuts, drained
¼ cup chopped green bell pepper
3 tablespoons chopped fresh parsley

2 tablespoons minced red onion
½ cup plain fat-free yogurt
1½ tablespoons lemon juice
¼ teaspoon freshly ground black pepper
1 head butter lettuce, cored and quartered
1 large tomato, cut into wedges

1. In a medium saucepan, boil 2½ cups of water. Slowly add the brown rice. Cover, and reduce the heat to low. Cook the rice for 45–50 minutes until tender. Do not continually stir the rice (this will cause it to become gummy). Just check it occasionally. 2. In a large salad bowl, combine all the ingredients except the lettuce and tomato wedges. Just before serving, line 4 plates with the lettuce, and spoon the salad on top of the lettuce. Garnish with the tomato wedges.

Per Serving

Calorie: 253 | fat: 2g | protein: 15g | carbs: 45g | sugars: 6g | fiber: 4g | sodium: 189mg

Greek Rice Salad

Prep time: 10 minutes | Cook time: 0 minutes | Serves 4

3 tablespoons fresh lemon juice
1½ tablespoons coconut nectar or pure maple syrup
1 tablespoon red wine vinegar
1 teaspoon sea salt
1 teaspoon Dijon mustard
¼ teaspoon allspice
½–1 teaspoon grated fresh garlic
Freshly ground black pepper to taste (optional)

4 cups cooked brown rice
1 cup chopped cucumber (seeds removed, if you prefer)
1 cup sliced grape or cherry tomatoes or chopped tomatoes (can substitute chopped red pepper)
½ cup sliced kalamata olives
½ tablespoon chopped fresh oregano
2 tablespoons chopped fresh dill

1. In a large bowl, whisk together the lemon juice, nectar or syrup, vinegar, salt, mustard, allspice, garlic, and pepper (if using). Add the rice, cucumber, tomatoes, olives, oregano, and dill, and stir to combine. Taste, and add extra salt or lemon juice, if desired. Serve as a side or as a hearty lunch over greens.

Per Serving

Calorie: 306 | fat: 4g | protein: 6g | carbs: 62g | sugars: 7g | fiber: 5g | sodium: 751mg

Strawberry-Spinach Salad

Prep time: 15 minutes | Cook time: 0 minutes | Serves 4

½ cup extra-virgin olive oil
¼ cup balsamic vinegar
1 tablespoon Worcestershire sauce
1 (10-ounce) package baby spinach
1 medium red onion, quartered
and sliced
1 cup strawberries, sliced
1 (6-ounce) container feta cheese, crumbled
1 cup slivered almonds, divided

1. In a large bowl, whisk together the olive oil, balsamic vinegar, and Worcestershire sauce. 2. Add the spinach, onion, strawberries, and feta cheese and mix until all the ingredients are coated. 3. Portion into 4 servings and top each with ¼ cup of slivered almonds. ·

Per Serving

Calorie: 417 | fat: 29g | protein: 24g | carbs: 19g | sugars: 7g | fiber: 7g | sodium: 542mg

Quinoa, Beet, and Greens Salad

Prep time: 15 minutes | Cook time: 25 minutes | Serves 2

For the vinaigrette
1 tablespoon extra-virgin olive oil
2 tablespoons red wine vinegar
1 garlic clove, chopped
Freshly ground black pepper, to season
For the salad
2 medium beets
1 small bunch fresh kale leaves, thoroughly washed, deveined, and dried
Extra-virgin olive oil cooking spray
⅓ cup dry quinoa
⅔ cup water
¼ cup chopped scallions
½ cup unsalted soy nuts

To make the vinaigrette In a large bowl, whisk together the olive oil, red wine vinegar, and garlic. Season with pepper. Set aside. To make the salad 1. Into a medium saucepan set over high heat, insert a steamer basket. Fill the pan with water to just below the bottom of the steamer. Cover and bring to a boil. 2. Add the beets. Cover and steam for 7 to 10 minutes, or until just tender. Remove from the steamer. Let sit until cool enough to handle. Peel and slice. Set aside. 3. Spray the kale leaves with cooking spray. Massage the leaves, breaking down the fibers so they're easier to chew. Chop finely. You should have 1 cup. 4. In a small saucepan set over high heat, mix together the quinoa and water. Bring to a boil. Reduce the heat to medium-low. Cover and simmer for about 15 minutes, or until the quinoa is tender and the liquid has been absorbed. Remove from the heat. 5. Immediately add half of the vinaigrette to the saucepan while fluffing the quinoa with a fork. Cover and refrigerate for at least 1 hour, or until completely cooled. Set aside the remaining vinaigrette. 6. Into the cooled quinoa, stir the chopped kale, scallions, soy nuts, sliced beets, and remaining vinaigrette. Toss lightly before serving.

Per Serving

Calorie: 461 | fat: 29g | protein: 14g | carbs: 41g | sugars: 7g | fiber: 9g | sodium: 100mg

Broccoli Slaw Crab Salad

Prep time: 15 minutes | Cook time: 0 minutes | Serves 4

⅔ cup mayonnaise
1 tablespoon freshly squeezed lime juice
1 teaspoon minced garlic
½ teaspoon freshly ground black pepper
1 (16-ounce) package broccoli slaw
2 (6-ounce) cans crabmeat, drained and flaked
1 small onion, diced
2 large celery stalks, chopped
1 large red bell pepper, seeded and chopped
Chopped fresh parsley, for garnish

1. In a large bowl, whisk together the mayonnaise, lime juice, garlic, and pepper until smooth. 2. Add the broccoli slaw, crab meat, onion, celery, and bell pepper and mix until all the ingredients are coated. 3. Garnish with parsley.

Per Serving

Calorie: 279 | fat: 14g | protein: 26g | carbs: 13g | sugars: 3g | fiber: 2g | sodium: 572mg

Rotisserie Chicken and Avocado Salad

Prep time: 15 minutes | Cook time: 0 minutes | Serves 4

½ cup plain Greek yogurt
1 tablespoon freshly squeezed lime juice
4 teaspoons chopped fresh cilantro
2 ripe avocados, peeled, pitted, and cubed
1 cup shredded rotisserie chicken meat
½ medium red onion, chopped
1 large tomato, diced
4 cups mixed leafy greens, divided

1. In a large bowl, stir together the Greek yogurt, lime juice, and cilantro to make a dressing. 2. Add the avocado, chicken, onion, and tomato and mix gently into the dressing. 3. Divide 1 cup of the greens into 4 bowls and top with the chicken salad.

Per Serving

Calorie: 269 | fat: 18g | protein: 14g | carbs: 16g | sugars: 5g | fiber: 9g | sodium: 93mg

Shaved Brussels Sprouts and Kale with Poppy Seed Dressing

Prep time: 20 minutes | Cook time: 0 minutes | Serves 4 to 6

1 pound Brussels sprouts, shaved
1 bunch kale, thinly shredded
4 scallions, both white and green parts, thinly sliced
4 ounces shredded Romano cheese
Poppy seed dressing
Kosher salt
Freshly ground black pepper

1. In a large bowl, toss together the Brussels sprouts, kale, scallions, and Romano cheese. Add the dressing to the greens and toss to combine. Season with salt and pepper to taste.

Per Serving

Calorie: 139 | fat: 7g | protein: 11g | carbs: 11g | sugars: 3g | fiber: 4g | sodium: 357mg

Chickpea Salad

Prep time: 15 minutes | Cook time: 0 minutes | Serves 4

½ cup bottled balsamic vinaigrette
1 (15-ounce) can chickpeas, rinsed and drained
1 cup cherry tomatoes
1 small red onion, quartered and sliced
2 large cucumbers, peeled and

cut into bite-size pieces
1 large zucchini, cut into bite-size pieces
1 (10-ounce) package frozen shelled edamame, steamed or microwaved
Chopped fresh parsley, for garnish

1. Pour the vinaigrette into a large bowl. Add the chickpeas, tomatoes, onion, cucumbers, zucchini, and edamame and toss until all the ingredients are coated. 2. Garnish with chopped parsley.

Per Serving

Calorie: 188 | fat: 4g | protein: 10g | carbs: 29g | sugars: 11g | fiber: 8g | sodium: 171mg

Cabbage Slaw Salad

Prep time: 15 minutes | Cook time: 0 minutes | Serves 6

2 cups finely chopped green cabbage
2 cups finely chopped red cabbage
2 cups grated carrots
3 scallions, both white and green parts, sliced

2 tablespoons extra-virgin olive oil
2 tablespoons rice vinegar
1 teaspoon honey
1 garlic clove, minced
¼ teaspoon salt

1. In a large bowl, toss together the green and red cabbage, carrots, and scallions. 2. In a small bowl, whisk together the oil, vinegar, honey, garlic, and salt. 3. Pour the dressing over the veggies and mix to thoroughly combine. 4. Serve immediately, or cover and chill for several hours before serving.

Per Serving

Calories: 80 | fat: 5g | protein: 1g | carbs: 10g | sugars: 6g | fiber: 3g | sodium: 126mg

Apple-Bulgur Salad

Prep time: 10 minutes | Cook time: 15 minutes | Serves 2

2 cups water
1 cup bulgur
1 teaspoon dried thyme
2 tablespoons extra-virgin olive oil
2 teaspoons cider vinegar

Kosher salt
Freshly ground black pepper
6 kale leaves, shredded
1 small apple, cored and diced
3 tablespoons sliced, toasted almonds

1. In a large saucepan, bring the water to a boil over high heat and remove it from the heat. Add the bulgur and thyme, cover, and allow the grain to rest for 7 to 15 minutes or until cooked through. 2. Meanwhile, in a large bowl, whisk together the extra-virgin olive oil and cider vinegar with a pinch of salt and pepper. Add the cooked bulgur, kale, apple, and almonds to the dressing

and toss to combine. Adjust the seasonings as desired. 3. Store any leftovers in an airtight container in the refrigerator for 3 to 5 days.

Per Serving

Calorie: 496 | fat: 22g | protein: 13g | carbs: 69g | sugars: 9g | fiber: 13g | sodium: 33mg

Romaine Lettuce Salad with Cranberry, Feta, and Beans

Prep time: 10 minutes | Cook time: 0 minutes | Serves 2

1 cup chopped fresh green beans
6 cups washed and chopped romaine lettuce
1 cup sliced radishes
2 scallions, sliced
¼ cup chopped fresh oregano
1 cup canned kidney beans, drained and rinsed

½ cup cranberries, fresh or frozen
¼ cup crumbled fat-free feta cheese
1 tablespoon extra-virgin olive oil
Salt, to season
Freshly ground black pepper, to season

1. In a microwave-safe dish, add the green beans and a small amount of water. Microwave on high for about 2 minutes, or until tender. 2. In a large bowl, toss together the romaine lettuce, radishes, scallions, and oregano. 3. Add the green beans, kidney beans, cranberries, feta cheese, and olive oil. Season with salt and pepper. Toss to coat. 4. Evenly divide between 2 plates and enjoy immediately.

Per Serving

Calorie: 271 | fat: 9g | protein: 16g | carbs: 36g | sugars: 10g | fiber: 13g | sodium: 573mg

Sweet Beet Grain Bowl

Prep time: 10 minutes | Cook time: 20 minutes | Serves 2

3 cups water
1 cup farro, rinsed
2 tablespoons extra-virgin olive oil
1 tablespoon honey
3 tablespoons cider vinegar
Pinch freshly ground black

pepper
4 small cooked beets, sliced
1 pear, cored and diced
6 cups mixed greens
⅓ cup pumpkin seeds, roasted
¼ cup ricotta cheese

1. In a medium saucepan, stir together the water and farro over high heat and bring to a boil. Reduce the heat to medium and simmer until the farro is tender, 15 to 20 minutes. Drain and rinse the farro under cold running water until cool. Set aside. 2. Meanwhile, in a small bowl, whisk together the extra-virgin olive oil, honey, and vinegar. Season with black pepper. 3. Evenly divide the farro between two bowls. Top each with the beets, pear, greens, pumpkin seeds, and ricotta. Drizzle the bowls with the dressing before serving and adjust the seasonings as desired.

Per Serving

Calorie: 750 | fat: 28g | protein: 21g | carbs: 104g | sugars: 18g | fiber: 12g | sodium: 174mg

Sunflower-Tuna-Cauliflower Salad

Prep time: 30 minutes | Cook time: 0 minutes | Serves 2

1 (5-ounce) can tuna packed in water, drained
½ cup plain nonfat Greek yogurt
1 teaspoon freshly squeezed lemon juice
1 teaspoon dried dill

1 scallion, chopped
¼ cup sunflower seeds
2 cups fresh chopped cauliflower florets
4 cups mixed salad greens, divided

1. In a medium bowl, mix together the tuna, yogurt, lemon juice, dill, scallion, and sunflower seeds. 2. Add the cauliflower. Toss gently to coat. 3. Cover and refrigerate for at least 2 hours before serving, stirring occasionally. 4. Serve half of the tuna mixture atop 2 cups of salad greens.

Per Serving

Calorie: 251 | fat: 11g | protein: 24g | carbs: 18g | sugars: 8g | fiber: 7g | sodium: 288mg

Power Salad

Prep time: 15 minutes | Cook time: 0 minutes | Serves 2

For the dressing
1 tablespoon extra-virgin olive oil
1 tablespoon freshly squeezed lemon juice
1 tablespoon balsamic vinegar
1 tablespoon chia seeds
1 teaspoon liquid stevia
Pinch salt
Freshly ground black pepper

For the salad
6 cups mixed baby greens
1 cup shelled edamame
1 cup chopped red cabbage
1 cup chopped red bell pepper
1 cup sliced fresh button mushrooms
½ cup sliced avocado
¼ cup sliced almonds
1 cup pea shoots, divided

To make the dressing 1. In a small bowl, whisk together the olive oil, lemon juice, balsamic vinegar, chia seeds, and stevia until well combined. Season with salt and pepper. To make the salad 2. In a large bowl, toss together the mixed greens, edamame, red cabbage, red bell pepper, mushrooms, avocado, and almonds. Drizzle the dressing over the salad. Toss again to coat well. 3. Divide the salad between 2 plates. Top each with ½ cup of pea shoots and serve.

Per Serving

Calorie: 449 | fat: 24g | protein: 22g | carbs: 47g | sugars: 11g | fiber: 16g | sodium: 86mg

Grilled Romaine with White Beans

Prep time: 5 minutes | Cook time: 8 minutes | Serves 4 to 6

3 tablespoons extra-virgin olive oil, divided
2 large heads romaine lettuce, halved lengthwise
2 tablespoons white miso

1 tablespoon water, plus more as needed
1 (15-ounce) can white beans, rinsed and drained
½ cup chopped fresh parsley

1. Preheat the grill or a grill pan. 2. Drizzle 2 tablespoons of extra-virgin olive oil over the cut sides of the romaine lettuce. 3. In a medium bowl, whisk the remaining 1 tablespoon of extra-virgin olive oil with the white miso and about 1 tablespoon of water. Add more water, if necessary, to reach a thin consistency. Add the white beans and parsley to the bowl, stir, adjust the seasonings as desired, and set aside. 4. When the grill is hot, put the romaine on the grill and cook for 1 to 2 minutes on each side or until lightly charred with grill marks. Remove the lettuce from the grill and repeat with remaining lettuce halves. Set the lettuce aside on a platter or individual plates and top with the beans.

Per Serving

Calorie: 242 | fat: 10g | protein: 11g | carbs: 31g | sugars: 4g | fiber: 11g | sodium: 282mg

Greek Island Potato Salad

Prep time: 5 minutes | Cook time: 35 minutes | Serves 10

⅓ cup extra-virgin olive oil
4 garlic cloves, minced
2 pounds red potatoes, cut into 1½-inch pieces (leave the skin on if you wish)
6 medium carrots, peeled, halved lengthwise, and cut into 1½-inch pieces

1 onion, chopped
16 ounces artichoke hearts packed in water, drained and cut in half
½ cup Kalamata olives, pitted and halved
¼ cup lemon juice

1. In a large skillet, heat the olive oil. Add the garlic, and sauté for 30 seconds. Add the potatoes, carrots, and onion; cook over medium heat for 25–30 minutes until vegetables are just tender. 2. Add the artichoke hearts, and cook for 3–5 minutes more. Remove from the heat, and stir in the olives and lemon juice. Season with a dash of salt and pepper. Transfer to a serving bowl, and serve warm.

Per Serving

Calorie: 178 | fat: 8g | protein: 4g | carbs: 25g | sugars: 4g | fiber: 6g | sodium: 134mg

Chinese Chicken Salad

Prep time: 10 minutes | Cook time: 0 minutes | Serves 4

2 cups cooked chicken, diced
1 cup finely chopped celery
1 cup shredded carrots
¼ cup crushed unsweetened pineapple, drained
2 tablespoons finely diced pimiento

Two 8-ounce cans water chestnuts, drained and chopped
2 scallions, chopped
⅓ cup low-fat mayonnaise
1 tablespoon light soy sauce
1 teaspoon lemon juice
8 large tomatoes, hollowed

1. In a large bowl, combine the chicken, celery, carrots, pineapple, pimiento, water chestnuts, and scallions. 2. In a separate bowl, combine the mayonnaise, soy sauce, and lemon juice. Mix well. Add the dressing to the salad, and toss. Cover, and chill in the refrigerator for 2–3 hours. 3. For each serving, place a small scoop of chicken salad into a hollowed-out tomato.

Per Serving

Calorie: 365 | fat: 16g | protein: 27g | carbs: 32g | sugars: 17g | fiber: 9g | sodium: 476mg

Grilled Hearts of Romaine with Buttermilk Dressing

Prep time: 5 minutes | Cook time: 5 minutes | Serves 4

For The Romaine
2 heads romaine lettuce, halved lengthwise
2 tablespoons extra-virgin olive oil
For the dressing
½ cup low-fat buttermilk

1 tablespoon extra-virgin olive oil
1 garlic clove, pressed
¼ bunch fresh chives, thinly chopped
1 pinch red pepper flakes

To make the romaine 1. Heat a grill pan over medium heat. 2. Brush each lettuce half with the olive oil, and place flat-side down on the grill. Grill for 3 to 5 minutes, or until the lettuce slightly wilts and develops light grill marks. To make the dressing 1. In a small bowl, whisk the buttermilk, olive oil, garlic, chives, and red pepper flakes together. 2. Drizzle 2 tablespoons of dressing over each romaine half, and serve.

Per Serving

Calorie: 157 | fat: 11g | protein: 5g | carbs: 12g | sugars: 5g | fiber: 7g | sodium: 84mg

Three Bean and Basil Salad

Prep time: 10 minutes | Cook time: 0 minutes | Serves 8

1 (15-ounce) can low-sodium chickpeas, drained and rinsed
1 (15-ounce) can low-sodium kidney beans, drained and rinsed
1 (15-ounce) can low-sodium white beans, drained and rinsed
1 red bell pepper, seeded and finely chopped
¼ cup chopped scallions, both

white and green parts
¼ cup finely chopped fresh basil
3 garlic cloves, minced
2 tablespoons extra-virgin olive oil
1 tablespoon red wine vinegar
1 teaspoon Dijon mustard
¼ teaspoon freshly ground black pepper

1. In a large mixing bowl, combine the chickpeas, kidney beans, white beans, bell pepper, scallions, basil, and garlic. Toss gently to combine. 2. In a small bowl, combine the olive oil, vinegar, mustard, and pepper. Toss with the salad. 3. Cover and refrigerate for an hour before serving, to allow the flavors to mix.

Per Serving

Calorie: 193 | fat: 5g | protein: 10g | carbs: 29g | sugars: 3g | fiber: 8g | sodium: 246mg

Chickpea "Tuna" Salad

Prep time: 15 minutes | Cook time: 0 minutes | Serves 2

2 cups canned chickpeas, drained and rinsed
½ cup plain nonfat Greek yogurt
2 small celery stalks, chopped

1 small cucumber, chopped
½ cup chopped red onion
2 tablespoons freshly squeezed lemon juice
1 tablespoon chia seeds

1 garlic clove, chopped
1 teaspoon minced fresh parsley
Salt, to season

Freshly ground black pepper, to season
2 large romaine lettuce leaves

1. In a medium bowl, roughly mash the chickpeas with the back of a fork. 2. Add the yogurt, celery, cucumber, red onion, lemon juice, chia seeds, garlic, and parsley. Mix well. Season with salt and pepper. 3. Place half of the chickpea mixture on each romaine lettuce leaf. Wrap and serve chilled or at room temperature.

Per Serving

Calorie: 293 | fat: 6g | protein: 17g | carbs: 46g | sugars: 14g | fiber: 13g | sodium: 401mg

Lentil-Apple Salad

Prep time: 30 minutes | Cook time: 0 minutes | Serves 2

1½ teaspoons apple cider vinegar
¼ teaspoon granulated stevia
Pinch salt
Freshly ground black pepper
1 tablespoon extra-virgin olive oil
1½ teaspoons water
1 cup finely diced peeled apple

½ cup finely diced plum tomatoes
1 (14.5-ounce) can lentils, drained and rinsed
1 tablespoon fresh thyme
1 tablespoon fresh tarragon
4 cups mixed salad greens, divided

1. In a large bowl, whisk together the apple cider vinegar, stevia, and salt until the stevia dissolves. Season with pepper. 2. Add the olive oil. Whisk until emulsified. 3. Add the water. Whisk again to loosen. 4. Add the apple and tomatoes. Toss to coat. Let sit for 15 minutes. 5. Add the lentils, thyme, and tarragon. Stir to combine. Let sit for 15 minutes more. 6. Plate 2 cups of salad greens and half of the lentil mixture for each serving.

Per Serving

Calorie: 230 | fat: 8g | protein: 11g | carbs: 37g | sugars: 13g | fiber: 8g | sodium: 54mg

First-of-the-Season Tomato, Peach, and Strawberry Salad

Prep time: 15 minutes | Cook time: 0 minutes | Serves 6

6 cups mixed spring greens
4 large ripe plum tomatoes, thinly sliced
4 large ripe peaches, pitted and thinly sliced
12 ripe strawberries, thinly sliced

½ Vidalia onion, thinly sliced
2 tablespoons white balsamic vinegar
2 tablespoons extra-virgin olive oil
Freshly ground black pepper

1. Put the greens in a large salad bowl, and layer the tomatoes, peaches, strawberries, and onion on top. 2. Dress with the vinegar and oil, toss together, and season with pepper.

Per Serving

Calorie: 122 | fat: 5g | protein: 3g | carbs: 19g | sugars: 14g | fiber: 4g | sodium: 20mg

Edamame and Walnut Salad

Prep time: 10 minutes | Cook time: 0 minutes | Serves 2

For the vinaigrette
2 tablespoons balsamic vinegar
1 tablespoon extra-virgin olive oil
1 teaspoon grated fresh ginger
½ teaspoon Dijon mustard
Pinch salt
Freshly ground black pepper, to season

For the salad
1 cup shelled edamame
½ cup shredded carrots
½ cup shredded red cabbage
½ cup walnut halves
6 cups prewashed baby spinach, divided

To make the vinaigrette: In a small bowl, whisk together the balsamic vinegar, olive oil, ginger, Dijon mustard, and salt. Season with pepper. Set aside. To make the salad
1. In a medium bowl, mix together the edamame, carrots, red cabbage, and walnuts. 2. Add the vinaigrette. Toss to coat. 3. Place 3 cups of spinach on each of 2 serving plates. 4. Top each serving with half of the dressed vegetables. 5. Enjoy immediately!

Per Serving

Calorie: 341 | fat: 26g | protein: 13g | carbs: 19g | sugars: 7g | fiber: 8g | sodium: 117mg

Zucchini, Carrot, and Fennel Salad

Prep time: 10 minutes | Cook time: 8 minutes | Serves ½ cup

2 medium carrots, peeled and julienned
1 medium zucchini, julienned
½ medium fennel bupounds, core removed and julienned
1 tablespoon fresh orange juice
2 tablespoons Dijon mustard
3 tablespoons extra-virgin olive oil
1 teaspoon white wine vinegar

½ teaspoon dried thyme
1 tablespoon finely minced parsley
1 teaspoon salt
¼ teaspoon freshly ground black pepper
¼ cup chopped walnuts
1 medium head romaine lettuce, washed and leaves separated

1. Place the carrots, zucchini, and fennel in a medium bowl; set aside. 2. In a medium bowl, combine the orange juice, mustard, olive oil, vinegar, thyme, parsley, salt, and pepper; mix well. 3. Pour the dressing over the vegetables and toss. Add the walnuts, and mix again. Refrigerate until ready to serve. 4. To serve, line a bowl or plates with lettuce leaves, and spoon ½ cup of salad on top.

Per Serving

Calorie: 201 | fat: 16g | protein: 5g | carbs: 14g | sugars: 6g | fiber: 6g | sodium: 285mg

Chapter 8 Desserts

Chocolate Almond Butter Fudge 81

Cherry Almond Cobbler 81

Basic Pie Crust 81

Peach Shortcake 81

Strawberry Chia Pudding 81

Mixed-Berry Cream Tart 82

Creamy Pineapple-Pecan Dessert
Squares 82

Mixed-Berry Snack Cake 82

5-Ingredient Chunky Cherry and Peanut
Butter Cookies 82

Pumpkin Cheesecake Smoothie 83

Dulce de Leche Fillo Cups 83

Oatmeal Cookies 83

Peanut Butter Fudge Brownies 83

Goat Cheese–Stuffed Pears 83

Chewy Chocolate-Oat Bars 84

Quick Yummy Peaches 84

Broiled Pineapple 84

Grilled Peach and Coconut Yogurt Bowls 84

Apple Crunch 84

Fried Apples 85

Low-Calorie, Fat-Free Whipped Cream 85

Mango Nice Cream 85

Oatmeal Chippers 85

Strawberry Cheesecake in a Jar 85

Crustless Key Lime Cheesecake 86

Peach and Almond Meal Fritters 86

Chocolate Baked Bananas 86

Coffee and Cream Pops 86

No-Added-Sugar Orange and Cream
Slushy 86

Chocolate Chip and Cranberry Cookies 87

Low-Fat Cream Cheese Frosting 87

Banana Pineapple Freeze 87

Double-Ginger Cookies 87

Simple Bread Pudding 87

Crumb Pie Shell 88

Blueberry Chocolate Clusters 88

Chipotle Black Bean Brownies 88

Baked Berry Cups with Crispy Cinnamon
Wedges 88

Chocolate Almond Butter Fudge

Prep time: 10 minutes | Cook time: 0 minutes | Makes 9 Pieces

2 ounces unsweetened baking chocolate	thickened cream only
½ cup almond butter	1 teaspoon vanilla extract
1 can full-fat coconut milk, refrigerated overnight,	4 (1-gram) packets stevia (or to taste)

1. Line a 9-inch square baking pan with parchment paper. 2. In a small saucepan over medium-low heat, heat the chocolate and almond butter, stirring constantly, until both are melted. Cool slightly. 3. In a medium bowl, combine the melted chocolate mixture with the cream from the coconut milk, vanilla, and stevia. Blend until smooth. Taste and adjust sweetness as desired. 4. Pour the mixture into the prepared pan, spreading with a spatula to smooth. Refrigerate for 3 hours. Cut into squares.

Per Serving1 piece:

Calories: 169 | fat: 11g | protein: 8g | carbs: 11g | sugars: 7g | fiber: 3g | sodium: 64mg

Cherry Almond Cobbler

Prep time: 10 minutes | Cook time: 25 minutes | Serves 4

2 cups water-packed sour cherries	¾ teaspoon baking powder
¼ teaspoon fresh lemon juice	1 tablespoon canola oil
⅛ teaspoon almond extract	¼ cup egg substitute
½ cup almond flour, sifted	2 tablespoons fat-free milk
⅛ teaspoon salt	¼ cup granulated sugar substitute (such as stevia)
¼ cup flaxseeds	

1. Preheat the oven to 425 degrees. Drain the cherries, reserving ⅔ cup of liquid, and place the cherries in a shallow 9-inch glass or porcelain cake pan. 2. In a small mixing bowl, combine the lemon juice, almond extract, and drained cherry liquid; mix well. Spoon over the cherries. 3. In a mixing bowl, combine the almond flour, flaxseeds, and baking powder. Mix thoroughly. Stir in the oil, egg substitute, milk, and sugar substitute, mixing well. 4. Spoon the mixture over the cherries, and bake at 425 degrees for 25–30 minutes or until the crust is golden brown.

Per Serving

Calories: 216 | fat: 14g | protein: 7g | carbs: 19g | sugars: 10g | fiber: 6g | sodium: 132mg

Basic Pie Crust

Prep time: 10 minutes | Cook time: 40 minutes | Serves 9

¾ cup cake flour	frozen for 15 minutes
½ teaspoon sugar	½ teaspoon white vinegar
1 teaspoon salt	2 tablespoons ice water
3 tablespoons canola oil,	

1. In a medium bowl, combine the flour, sugar, and salt. Stir in the oil and mix until the mixture is the size of small peas. 2. Add the vinegar and ice water and mix with a fork until the dough starts to hold together. Gather into a ball, wrap, and refrigerate at least 30 minutes before rolling out. 3. Roll out the pie crust to fit an 8- or 9-inch pie dish. Lay the rolled dough in the pan without stretching it, and crimp the edges. 4. If the recipe requires a baked pie crust, preheat the oven to 425 degrees. Prick the crust with a fork, and lay a piece of parchment or wax paper in the pie shell. Pour in enough dried beans to cover the bottom (this prevents the crust from bubbling up while baking). Bake for 8 minutes or until golden brown.

Per Serving

Calories: 84 | fat: 5g | protein: 1g | carbs: 9g | sugars: 0g | fiber: 0g | sodium: 129mg

Peach Shortcake

Prep time: 10 minutes | Cook time: 30 minutes | Serves 8

2½ cups sliced fresh peaches	½ teaspoon almond extract
½ cup slivered almonds	½ teaspoon cinnamon
1½ tablespoons plus 1 teaspoon granulated sugar substitute (such as stevia), divided	1 cup whole-wheat flour
	2 teaspoons baking powder
	2 tablespoons canola oil
	¼ cup egg substitute
	¼ cup fat-free milk

1. Preheat the oven to 400 degrees. 2. Lightly spray an 8-x-8-x-2-inch baking pan with nonstick cooking spray. Arrange the peaches and almonds in the bottom of the dish. 3. In a small bowl, mix together 1 teaspoon of the sugar substitute, the almond extract, and the cinnamon; sprinkle over the peaches, and set aside. 4. In a medium bowl, combine the flour, baking powder, and the remaining 1½ tablespoons of sugar substitute; mix well. 5. Add the oil, egg substitute, and milk to the dry ingredients; mix until smooth. Spread evenly over the peaches, and bake for 25–30 minutes or until the top is golden brown. Remove from the oven, invert onto a serving plate, and serve.

Per Serving

Calories: 110 | fat: 4g | protein: 3g | carbs: 16g | sugars: 5g | fiber: 3g | sodium: 22mg

Strawberry Chia Pudding

Prep time: 5 minutes | Cook time: 0 minutes | Serves 2

1½ cups frozen whole strawberries	1 teaspoon lemon juice
3 tablespoons white chia seeds	Pinch of sea salt
1 tablespoon coconut nectar or pure maple syrup	½ cup + 2–3 tablespoons plain low-fat nondairy milk

1. In a blender, combine the strawberries, chia seeds, nectar or syrup, lemon juice, salt, and ½ cup plus 2 tablespoons of the milk. Puree until the seeds are fully pulverized and the pudding begins to thicken. (It will thicken more as it cools.) Add the extra 1 tablespoon milk if needed to blend. Transfer the mixture to a large bowl or dish and refrigerate until chilled, about an hour or more. (It will thicken more with chilling, but really can be eaten right away.)

Per Serving

Calorie: 185 | fat: 5g | protein: 4g | carbs: 33g | sugars: 16g | fiber: 9g | sodium: 182mg

Mixed-Berry Cream Tart

Prep time: 20 minutes | Cook time: 0 minutes | Serves 8

2 cups sliced fresh strawberries	1 package (8 ounce) fat-free cream cheese
½ cup boiling water	¼ cup sugar
1 box (4-serving size) sugar-free strawberry gelatin	¼ teaspoon almond extract
3 pouches (1.5 ounces each) roasted almond crunchy granola bars (from 8.9-ounce box)	1 cup fresh blueberries
	1 cup fresh raspberries
	Fat-free whipped topping, if desired

1. In small bowl, crush 1 cup of the strawberries with pastry blender or fork. Reserve remaining 1 cup strawberries. 2. In medium bowl, pour boiling water over gelatin; stir about 2 minutes or until gelatin is completely dissolved. Stir crushed strawberries into gelatin. Refrigerate 20 minutes. 3. Meanwhile, leaving granola bars in pouches, crush granola bars with rolling pin. Sprinkle crushed granola in bottom of 9-inch ungreased glass pie plate, pushing crumbs up side of plate to make crust. 4. In small bowl, beat cream cheese, sugar and almond extract with electric mixer on medium-high speed until smooth. Drop by teaspoonfuls over crushed granola; gently spread to cover bottom of crust. 5. Gently fold blueberries, raspberries and remaining 1 cup strawberries into gelatin mixture. Spoon over cream cheese mixture. Refrigerate about 3 hours or until firm. Serve topped with whipped topping.

Per Serving

Calorie: 170 | fat: 3g | protein: 8g | carbs: 27g | sugars: 17g | fiber: 3g | sodium: 340mg

Creamy Pineapple-Pecan Dessert Squares

Prep time: 25 minutes | Cook time: 0 minutes | Serves 18

¾ cup boiling water	¼ cup chopped pecans
1 package (4-serving size) lemon sugar-free gelatin	3 tablespoons butter or margarine, melted
1 cup unsweetened pineapple juice	1 package (8 ounces) fat-free cream cheese
1½ cups graham cracker crumbs	1 container (8 ounces) fat-free sour cream
½ cup sugar	1 can (8 ounces) crushed pineapple, undrained
¼ cup shredded coconut	

1. In large bowl, pour boiling water over gelatin; stir about 2 minutes or until gelatin is completely dissolved. Stir in pineapple juice. Refrigerate about 30 minutes or until mixture is syrupy and just beginning to thicken. 2. Meanwhile, in 13x9-inch (3-quart) glass baking dish, toss cracker crumbs, ¼ cup of the sugar, the coconut, pecans and melted butter until well mixed. Reserve ½ cup crumb mixture for topping. Press remaining mixture in bottom of dish. 3. In medium bowl, beat cream cheese, sour cream and remaining ¼ cup sugar with electric mixer on medium speed until smooth; set aside. 4. Beat gelatin mixture with electric mixer on low speed until foamy; beat on high speed until light and fluffy (mixture will look like beaten egg whites). Beat in cream cheese mixture just until mixed.

Gently stir in pineapple (with liquid). Pour into crust-lined dish; smooth top. Sprinkle reserved ½ cup crumb mixture over top. Refrigerate about 4 hours or until set. For servings, cut into 6 rows by 3 rows.

Per Serving

Calorie: 120 | fat: 4.5g | protein: 3g | carbs: 18g | sugars: 11g | fiber: 0g | sodium: 180mg

Mixed-Berry Snack Cake

Prep time: 15 minutes | Cook time: 28 to 33 minutes | Serves 8

¼ cup low-fat granola	½ teaspoon baking soda
½ cup buttermilk	½ teaspoon ground cinnamon
⅓ cup packed brown sugar	⅛ teaspoon salt
2 tablespoons canola oil	1 cup mixed fresh berries (such as blueberries, raspberries and blackberries)
1 teaspoon vanilla	
1 egg	
1 cup whole wheat flour	

1. Heat oven to 350°F. Spray 8- or 9-inch round pan with cooking spray. Place granola in resealable food-storage plastic bag; seal bag and slightly crush with rolling pin or meat mallet. Set aside. 2 In large bowl, stir buttermilk, brown sugar, oil, vanilla and egg until smooth. Stir in flour, baking soda, cinnamon and salt just until moistened. Gently fold in half of the berries. Spoon into pan. Sprinkle with remaining berries and the granola. 3 Bake 28 to 33 minutes or until golden brown and top springs back when touched in center. Cool in pan on cooling rack 10 minutes. Serve warm.

Per Serving

Calorie: 160 | fat: 5g | protein: 3g | carbs: 26g | sugars: 12g | fiber: 1g | sodium: 140mg

5-Ingredient Chunky Cherry and Peanut Butter Cookies

Prep time: 5 minutes | Cook time: 10 to 12 minutes | Makes 12 cookies

1 cup (240 g) all-natural peanut butter	1 large egg, beaten
¼ cup (60 ml) pure maple syrup	1 cup (80 g) gluten-free rolled or quick oats
	½ cup (80 g) dried cherries

1. Preheat the oven to 350°F (177°C). Line a large baking sheet with parchment paper. 2. In a large bowl, whisk together the peanut butter, maple syrup, and egg. Add the oats and cherries, and mix until the ingredients are combined. 3. Chill the dough for 10 to 15 minutes. 4. Use a cookie scoop to scoop balls of the dough onto the prepared baking sheet. 5. Using a fork, gently flatten the dough balls into your desired shape (the cookies will not change shape much during baking). Bake the cookies for 10 to 12 minutes, until they are lightly golden on top. 6. Remove the cookies from the oven and let them cool for 5 minutes before transferring them to a wire rack.

Per Serving

Calorie: 198 | fat: 12g | protein: 7g | carbs: 19g | sugars: 11g | fiber: 3g | sodium: 13mg

Pumpkin Cheesecake Smoothie

Prep time: 10 minutes | Cook time: 0 minutes | Serves 1

2 tablespoons cream cheese, at room temperature
½ cup canned pumpkin purée (not pumpkin pie mix)

1 cup almond milk
1 teaspoon pumpkin pie spice
½ cup crushed ice

1. In a blender, combine all of the ingredients. Blend until smooth.

Per Serving

Calories: 230 | fat: 11g | protein: 11g | carbs: 25g | sugars: 16g | fiber: 4g | sodium: 216mg

Dulce de Leche Fillo Cups

Prep time: 15 minutes | Cook time: 0 minutes | Serves 15

2 ounce ⅓-less-fat cream cheese (Neufchâtel), softened
2 tablespoons dulce de leche (caramel) syrup
1 tablespoon reduced-fat sour

cream
1 package frozen mini fillo shells (15 shells)
⅓ cup sliced fresh strawberries
2 tablespoons diced mango

1. In medium bowl, beat cream cheese with electric mixer on low speed until creamy. Beat in dulce de leche syrup and sour cream until blended. 2. Spoon cream cheese mixture into each fillo shell. Top each with strawberries and mango.

Per Serving

Calorie: 40 | fat: 2g | protein: 0g | carbs: 4g | sugars: 2g | fiber: 0g | sodium: 35mg

Oatmeal Cookies

Prep time: 5 minutes | Cook time: 15 minutes | Serves 16

¾ cup almond flour
¾ cup old-fashioned oats
¼ cup shredded unsweetened coconut
1 teaspoon baking powder
1 teaspoon ground cinnamon

¼ teaspoon salt
¼ cup unsweetened applesauce
1 large egg
1 tablespoon pure maple syrup
2 tablespoons coconut oil, melted

1. Preheat the oven to 350°F. 2. In a medium mixing bowl, combine the almond flour, oats, coconut, baking powder, cinnamon, and salt, and mix well. 3. In another medium bowl, combine the applesauce, egg, maple syrup, and coconut oil, and mix. Stir the wet mixture into the dry mixture. 4. Form the dough into balls a little bigger than a tablespoon and place on a baking sheet, leaving at least 1 inch between them. Bake for 12 minutes until the cookies are just browned. Remove from the oven and let cool for 5 minutes. 5. Using a spatula, remove the cookies and cool on a rack.

Per Serving

Calorie: 76 | fat: 6g | protein: 2g | carbs: 5g | sugars: 1g | fiber: 1g | sodium: 57mg

Peanut Butter Fudge Brownies

Prep time: 5 minutes | Cook time: 15 minutes | Makes 12 brownies

Cooking oil spray, as needed
1 cup (80 g) gluten-free rolled oats
½ cup (48 g) almond flour
1 cup (194 g) canned low-sodium black beans, drained and rinsed
¼ cup (60 ml) cooking oil of choice
1½ teaspoons (8 ml) pure vanilla extract
¼ teaspoons baking soda

1 teaspoon baking powder
¼ teaspoons sea salt
1 teaspoon ground cinnamon
⅓ cup (32 g) unsweetened cocoa powder
½ cup (120 ml) pure maple syrup
¼ cup (45 g) dairy-free dark chocolate chips
2 tablespoons (30 g) all-natural peanut butter (see Tip)

1. Preheat the oven to 350°F (177°C). Spray an 8 x 8–inch (20 x 20–cm) baking pan with the cooking oil spray. 2. In a food processor, combine the oats, almond flour, beans, oil, vanilla, baking soda, baking powder, sea salt, cinnamon, cocoa powder, and maple syrup. Process the ingredients for about 1 minute, until the batter is smooth. You may need to stop the food processor once and scrape down the sides. 3. Carefully remove the food processor's blade and stir in the chocolate chips by hand. 4. Spread the batter into the prepared baking pan. Drizzle the peanut butter over the top of the batter. 5. Bake the brownies for 15 minutes, until a toothpick inserted into the center comes out clean. Let the brownies cool completely in the pan on a wire rack.

Per Serving 1 brownie:

Calorie: 170 | fat: 10g | protein: 3g | carbs: 19g | sugars: 11g | fiber: 2g | sodium: 52mg

Goat Cheese–Stuffed Pears

Prep time: 6 minutes | Cook time: 2 minutes | Serves 4

2 ounces goat cheese, at room temperature
2 teaspoons pure maple syrup
2 ripe, firm pears, halved

lengthwise and cored
2 tablespoons chopped pistachios, toasted

1. Pour 1 cup of water into the electric pressure cooker and insert a wire rack or trivet. 2. In a small bowl, combine the goat cheese and maple syrup. 3. Spoon the goat cheese mixture into the cored pear halves. Place the pears on the rack inside the pot, cut-side up. 4. Close and lock the lid of the pressure cooker. Set the valve to sealing. 5. Cook on high pressure for 2 minutes. 6. When the cooking is complete, hit Cancel and quick release the pressure. 7. Once the pin drops, unlock and remove the lid. 8. Using tongs, carefully transfer the pears to serving plates. 9. Sprinkle with pistachios and serve immediately.

Per Serving (½ pear):

Calories: 120 | fat: 5g | protein: 4g | carbs: 17g | sugars: 11g | fiber: 3g | sodium: 54mg

Chewy Chocolate-Oat Bars

Prep time: 20 minutes | Cook time: 30 minutes | Makes 16 bars

¾ cup semisweet chocolate chips
⅓ cup fat-free sweetened condensed milk (from 14-ounce can)
1 cup whole wheat flour
½ cup quick-cooking oats
½ teaspoon baking powder
½ teaspoon baking soda
¼ teaspoon salt

¼ cup fat-free egg product or 1 egg
¾ cup packed brown sugar
¼ cup canola oil
1 teaspoon vanilla
2 tablespoons quick-cooking oats
2 teaspoons butter or margarine, softened

1. Eat oven to 350°F. Spray 8-inch or 9-inch square pan with cooking spray. 2. in 1-quart saucepan, heat chocolate chips and milk over low heat, stirring frequently, until chocolate is melted and mixture is smooth. Remove from heat. 3. In large bowl, mix flour, ½ cup oats, the baking powder, baking soda and salt; set aside. In medium bowl, stir egg product, brown sugar, oil and vanilla with fork until smooth. Stir into flour mixture until blended. Reserve ½ cup dough in small bowl for topping. 4. Pat remaining dough in pan (if dough is sticky, spray fingers with cooking spray or dust with flour). Spread chocolate mixture over dough. Add 2 tablespoons oats and the butter to reserved ½ cup dough; mix with pastry blender or fork until well mixed. Place small pieces of mixture evenly over chocolate mixture. 5. Bake 20 to 25 minutes or until top is golden and firm. Cool completely, about 1 hour 30 minutes. For bars, cut into 4 rows by 4 rows.

Per Serving 1 Bar:

Calorie: 180 | fat: 7g | protein: 3g | carbs: 27g | sugars: 18g | fiber: 1g | sodium: 115mg

Quick Yummy Peaches

Prep time: 20 minutes | Cook time: 20 minutes | Serves 8

⅓ cup buttermilk baking mix
⅔ cup dry quick oats
¼ cup brown sugar
Brown sugar substitute to equal 2 tablespoons sugar

1 teaspoon cinnamon
4 cups sliced peaches, canned or fresh
½ cup peach juice or water
1 cup water

1. Mix together baking mix, oats, brown sugar, brown sugar substitute, and cinnamon. Mix in the peaches and peach juice. 2. Pour mixture into a 1.6-quart baking dish. Cover with foil. 3. Place the trivet into your Instant Pot and pour in 1 cup of water. Place a foil sling on top of the trivet, then place the baking dish on top. 4. Secure the lid and make sure lid is set to sealing. Press Manual and set for 10 minutes. 5. When cook time is up, let the pressure release naturally for 10 minutes, then release any remaining pressure manually. Carefully remove the baking dish by using hot pads to lift the foil sling. Uncover and let cool for about 20–30 minutes.

Per Serving

Calories: 131 | fat: 1g | protein: 2g | carbs: 29g | sugars: 20g | fiber: 3g | sodium: 76mg

Broiled Pineapple

Prep time: 5 minutes | Cook time: 5 minutes | Serves 4

4 large slices fresh pineapple
2 tablespoons canned coconut milk

2 tablespoons unsweetened shredded coconut
¼ teaspoon sea salt

1. Preheat the oven broiler on high. 2. On a rimmed baking sheet, arrange the pineapple in a single layer. Brush lightly with the coconut milk and sprinkle with the coconut. 3. Broil until the pineapple begins to brown, 3 to 5 minutes. 4. Sprinkle with the sea salt.

Per Serving

Calories: 110 | fat: 3g | protein: 1g | carbs: 23g | sugars: 15g | fiber: 3g | sodium: 16mg

Grilled Peach and Coconut Yogurt Bowls

Prep time: 5 minutes | Cook time: 10 minutes | Serves 4

2 peaches, halved and pitted
½ cup plain nonfat Greek yogurt
1 teaspoon pure vanilla extract
¼ cup unsweetened dried

coconut flakes
2 tablespoons unsalted pistachios, shelled and broken into pieces

1. Preheat the broiler to high. Arrange the rack in the closest position to the broiler. 2. In a shallow pan, arrange the peach halves, cut-side up. Broil for 6 to 8 minutes until browned, tender, and hot. 3. In a small bowl, mix the yogurt and vanilla. 4. Spoon the yogurt into the cavity of each peach half. 5. Sprinkle 1 tablespoon of coconut flakes and 1½ teaspoons of pistachios over each peach half. Serve warm.

Per Serving

Calories: 102 | fat: 5g | protein: 5g | carbs: 11g | sugars: 8g | fiber: 2g | sodium: 12mg

Apple Crunch

Prep time: 13 minutes | Cook time: 2 minutes | Serves 4

3 apples, peeled, cored, and sliced (about 1½ pounds)
1 teaspoon pure maple syrup
1 teaspoon apple pie spice or

ground cinnamon
¼ cup unsweetened apple juice, apple cider, or water
¼ cup low-sugar granola

1. In the electric pressure cooker, combine the apples, maple syrup, apple pie spice, and apple juice. 2. Close and lock the lid of the pressure cooker. Set the valve to sealing. 3. Cook on high pressure for 2 minutes. 4. When the cooking is complete, hit Cancel and quick release the pressure. 5. Once the pin drops, unlock and remove the lid. 6. Spoon the apples into 4 serving bowls and sprinkle each with 1 tablespoon of granola.

Per Serving

Calories: 103 | fat: 1g | protein: 1g | carbs: 26g | sugars: 18g | fiber: 4g | sodium: 13mg

Fried Apples

Prep time: 5 minutes | Cook time: 15 minutes | Serves 6 to 8

4 Pink Lady apples, quartered
¼ cup erythritol or other

brown sugar replacement

1. In a small mixing bowl, toss the apples in the erythritol. Working in batches, place in the basket of an air fryer. 2. Set the air fryer to 390°F, close, and cook for 15 minutes. 3. Once cooking is complete, transfer the apples to a plate. Repeat until no apples remain.

Per Serving

Calories: 50 | fat: 0g | protein: 0g | carbs: 13g | sugars: 9g | fiber: 2g | sodium: 5mg

Low-Calorie, Fat-Free Whipped Cream

Prep time: 5 minutes | Cook time: 5 minutes | Serves 8

2 tablespoons water
1 teaspoon unflavored gelatin
½ cup fat-free powdered milk

1 teaspoon vanilla extract
1 cup ice water
½ teaspoon agave nectar

1. In a small skillet, add the water; sprinkle gelatin on top. 2. After the gelatin has soaked in, stir over low heat until clear; cool. In a large mixing bowl, combine the milk, vanilla, ice water, and agave nectar; mix well. 3. Add the gelatin mixture, and whip until fluffy with a wire whisk or electric beaters. Refrigerate the whipped cream until ready to use.

Per Serving

Calories: 10 | fat: 0g | protein: 1g | carbs: 1g | sugars: 1g | fiber: 0g | sodium: 11mg

Mango Nice Cream

Prep time: 10 minutes | Cook time: 0 minutes | Serves 4

2 cups frozen mango chunks
1 cup frozen, sliced, overripe banana (can use room temperature, but must be overripe)
Pinch of sea salt

½ teaspoon pure vanilla extract
¼ cup + 1–2 tablespoons low-fat nondairy milk
2–3 tablespoons coconut nectar or pure maple syrup (optional)

1. In a food processor or high-speed blender, combine the mango, banana, salt, vanilla, and ¼ cup of the milk. Pulse to get things moving, and then puree, adding the remaining 1 to 2 tablespoons milk if needed. Taste, and add the nectar or syrup, if desired. Serve, or transfer to an airtight container and freeze for an hour or more to set more firmly before serving.

Per Serving

Calorie: 116 | fat: 0.5g | protein: 1g | carbs: 29g | sugars: 18g | fiber: 2g | sodium: 81mg

Oatmeal Chippers

Prep time: 10 minutes | Cook time: 11 minutes | Makes 20 chippers

3–3½ tablespoons almond butter (or tigernut butter, for nut-free)
¼ cup pure maple syrup
¼ cup brown rice syrup
2 teaspoons pure vanilla extract
1⅓ cups oat flour

1 cup + 2 tablespoons rolled oats
1½ teaspoons baking powder
½ teaspoon cinnamon
¼ teaspoon sea salt
2–3 tablespoons sugar-free nondairy chocolate chips

1. Preheat the oven to 350°F. Line a baking sheet with parchment paper. 2. In the bowl of a mixer, combine the almond butter, maple syrup, brown rice syrup, and vanilla. Using the paddle attachment, mix on low speed for a couple of minutes, until creamy. Turn off the mixer and add the flour, oats, baking powder, cinnamon, salt, and chocolate chips. Mix on low speed until incorporated. Place 1½-tablespoon mounds on the prepared baking sheet, spacing them 1" to 2" apart, and flatten slightly. Bake for 11 minutes, or until just set to the touch. Remove from the oven, let cool on the pan for just a minute, and then transfer the cookies to a cooling rack.

Per Serving

Calorie: 90 | fat: 2g | protein: 2g | carbs: 16g | sugars: 4g | fiber: 2g | sodium: 75mg

Strawberry Cheesecake in a Jar

Prep time: 5 minutes | Cook time: 0 minutes | Serves 8

½ cup (55 g) raw cashews
¼ cup (60 g) all-natural peanut butter
2 tablespoons (12 g) almond flour
1 large pitted Medjool date
1 cup (200 g) coarsely chopped strawberries, plus more as needed

8 ounces (227 g) cream cheese
½ cup (100 g) plain nonfat Greek yogurt
¼ cup (60 ml) pure maple syrup
Zest of 1 medium lemon, plus more as needed
1 tablespoon (15 ml) pure vanilla extract

1. In a food processor, combine the cashews, peanut butter, almond flour, and Medjool date. Process the ingredients until a dough forms. 2. Divide the dough among eight (8-ounce [227-ml]) mason jars. Press the dough down into each jar to make a crust. 3. Divide the strawberries among the jars on top of the crusts. 4. In a food processor or high-power blender, combine the cream cheese, yogurt, maple syrup, lemon zest, and vanilla. Process the ingredients until they are smooth. 5. Divide the cheesecake mixture evenly among the jars, tapping them gently on the counter to shake out all the air bubbles. 6. Top the cheesecakes with additional strawberries and lemon zest if desired. 7. Refrigerate the cheesecakes for at least 2 hours or overnight before serving.

Per Serving

Calorie: 253 | fat: 18g | protein: 7g | carbs: 17g | sugars: 12g | fiber: 2g | sodium: 115mg

Chapter 8 Desserts | 85

Crustless Key Lime Cheesecake

Prep time: 15 minutes | Cook time: 35 minutes | Serves 8

Nonstick cooking spray
16 ounces light cream cheese (Neufchâtel), softened
⅔ cup granulated erythritol sweetener
¼ cup unsweetened Key lime juice (I like Nellie & Joe's Famous Key West Lime Juice)
½ teaspoon vanilla extract
¼ cup plain Greek yogurt
1 teaspoon grated lime zest
2 large eggs
Whipped cream, for garnish (optional)

1. Spray a 7-inch springform pan with nonstick cooking spray. Line the bottom and partway up the sides of the pan with foil. 2. Put the cream cheese in a large bowl. Use an electric mixer to whip the cream cheese until smooth, about 2 minutes. Add the erythritol, lime juice, vanilla, yogurt, and zest, and blend until smooth. Stop the mixer and scrape down the sides of the bowl with a rubber spatula. With the mixer on low speed, add the eggs, one at a time, blending until just mixed. (Don't overbeat the eggs.) 3. Pour the mixture into the prepared pan. Drape a paper towel over the top of the pan, not touching the cream cheese mixture, and tightly wrap the top of the pan in foil. (Your goal here is to keep out as much moisture as possible.) 4. Pour 1 cup of water into the electric pressure cooker. 5. Place the foil-covered pan onto the wire rack and carefully lower it into the pot. 6. Close and lock the lid of the pressure cooker. Set the valve to sealing. 7. Cook on high pressure for 35 minutes. 8. When the cooking is complete, hit Cancel. Allow the pressure to release naturally for 20 minutes, then quick release any remaining pressure. 9. Once the pin drops, unlock and remove the lid. 10. Using the handles of the wire rack, carefully transfer the pan to a cooling rack. Cool to room temperature, then refrigerate for at least 3 hours. 11. When ready to serve, run a thin rubber spatula around the rim of the cheesecake to loosen it, then remove the ring. 12. Slice into wedges and serve with whipped cream (if using).

Per Serving

Calories: 127 | fat: 2g | protein: 11g | carbs: 17g | sugars: 14g | fiber: 0g | sodium: 423mg

Peach and Almond Meal Fritters

Prep time: 15 minutes | Cook time: 15 minutes | Serves 7

4 ripe bananas, peeled
2 cups chopped peaches
1 medium egg
2 medium egg whites
¾ cup almond meal
¼ teaspoon almond extract

1. In a large bowl, mash the bananas and peaches together with a fork or potato masher. 2. Blend in the egg and egg whites. 3. Stir in the almond meal and almond extract. 4. Working in batches, place ¼-cup portions of the batter into the basket of an air fryer. 5. Set the air fryer to 390°F, close, and cook for 12 minutes. 6. Once cooking is complete, transfer the fritters to a plate. Repeat until no batter remains.

Per Serving

Calories: 150 | fat: 6g | protein: 5g | carbs: 22g | sugars: 12g | fiber: 4g | sodium: 25mg

Chocolate Baked Bananas

Prep time: 10 minutes | Cook time: 8 to 10 minutes | Serves 5

4–5 large ripe bananas, sliced lengthwise
2 tablespoons coconut nectar or pure maple syrup
1 tablespoon cocoa powder
Couple pinches sea salt
2 tablespoons nondairy chocolate chips (for finishing)
1 tablespoon chopped pecans, walnuts, almonds, or pumpkin seeds (for finishing)

1. Line a baking sheet with parchment paper and preheat oven to 450°F. Place bananas on the parchment. In a bowl, mix the coconut nectar or maple syrup with the cocoa powder and salt. Stir well to fully combine. Drizzle the chocolate mixture over the bananas. Bake for 8 to 10 minutes, until bananas are softened and caramelized. Sprinkle on chocolate chips and nuts, and serve.

Per Serving

Calorie: 146 | fat: 3g | protein: 2g | carbs: 34g | sugars: 18g | fiber: 4g | sodium: 119mg

Coffee and Cream Pops

Prep time: 10 minutes | Cook time: 5 minutes | Serves 4

2 teaspoons espresso powder (or to taste)
2 cups canned coconut milk
½ teaspoon vanilla extract
½ teaspoon cinnamon
3 (1-gram) packets stevia

1. In a medium saucepan over medium-low heat, heat all of the ingredients, stirring constantly, until the espresso powder is completely dissolved, about 5 minutes. 2. Pour the mixture into 4 ice pop molds. Freeze for 6 hours before serving.

Per Serving

Calories: 230 | fat: 24g | protein: 2g | carbs: 1g | sugars: 0g | fiber: 1g | sodium: 16mg

No-Added-Sugar Orange and Cream Slushy

Prep time: 5 minutes | Cook time: 0 minutes | Serves 2

½ cup (120 ml) unsweetened vanilla almond milk
½ cup (100 g) plain whole-milk yogurt
2 small oranges, peeled, seeds and pith removed, and frozen
1 small banana, frozen
1 teaspoon pure vanilla extract
2 tablespoons (10 g) unsweetened coconut flakes
1 tablespoon (12 g) chia seeds

1. In a high-power blender, combine the almond milk, yogurt, oranges, banana, vanilla, coconut flakes, and chia seeds. Blend the ingredients for 30 to 45 seconds, until a slushy consistency is reached.

Per Serving

Calorie: 203 | fat: 7g | protein: 8g | carbs: 29g | sugars: 17g | fiber: 7g | sodium: 67mg

Chocolate Chip and Cranberry Cookies

Prep time: 15 minutes | Cook time: 10 minutes | Serves 15

¼ cup canola oil
¼ cup granulated sugar substitute (such as stevia)
1 egg white
1 teaspoon vanilla
1 cup almond flour

¼ teaspoon baking soda
¼ teaspoon salt
4 tablespoons semisweet chocolate mini morsels
½ cup dried cranberries
½ cup chopped walnuts

1. Preheat the oven to 375 degrees. 2. In a medium bowl, cream the oil and sugar substitute, Beat in the egg white and vanilla; mix thoroughly. 3. In a sifter, combine the flour, baking soda, and salt. Sift the dry ingredients into the creamed mixture, and mix well. Stir in the chocolate mini morsels, cranberries, and walnuts. 4. Lightly spray cookie sheets with nonstick cooking spray. Drop teaspoonfuls of dough onto the cookie sheet. Place in the freezer for 10 minutes to chill. 5. Bake at 375 degrees for 8–10 minutes. Remove the cookies from the oven, and cool them on racks.

Per Serving

Calories: 119 | fat: 10g | protein: 2g | carbs: 5g | sugars: 3g | fiber: 2g | sodium: 45mg

Low-Fat Cream Cheese Frosting

Prep time: 5 minutes | Cook time: 0 minutes | Serves 8

3 cups fat-free ricotta cheese
1⅓ cups plain fat-free yogurt, strained overnight in cheesecloth over a bowl set in the refrigerator

2 cups low-fat cottage cheese
⅓ cup fructose
3 tablespoons evaporated fat-free milk

1. In a large bowl, combine all the ingredients; beat well with electric beaters until slightly stiff. 2. Place frosting in a covered container, and refrigerate until ready to use (this frosting can be refrigerated for up to 1 week).

Per Serving

Calories: 209 | fat: 7g | protein: 24g | carbs: 9g | sugars: 7g | fiber: 1g | sodium: 594mg

Banana Pineapple Freeze

Prep time: 30 minutes | Cook time: 0 minutes | Serves 12

2 cups mashed ripe bananas
2 cups unsweetened orange juice
2 tablespoon fresh lemon juice

1 cup unsweetened crushed pineapple, undrained
½ teaspoon ground cinnamon

1. In a food processor, combine all ingredients, and process until smooth and creamy. 2. Pour the mixture into a 9-x-9-x-2-inch baking dish, and freeze overnight or until firm. Serve chilled.

Per Serving

Calories: 60 | fat: 0g | protein: 1g | carbs: 15g | sugars: 9g | fiber: 1g | sodium: 1mg

Double-Ginger Cookies

Prep time: 45 minutes | Cook time: 8 to 10 minutes | Makes 5 dozen cookies

¾ cup sugar
¼ cup butter or margarine, softened
1 egg or ¼ cup fat-free egg product
¼ cup molasses
1¾ cups all-purpose flour
1 teaspoon baking soda

½ teaspoon ground cinnamon
½ teaspoon ground ginger
¼ teaspoon ground cloves
¼ teaspoon salt
¼ cup sugar
¼ cup orange marmalade
2 tablespoons finely chopped crystallized ginger

1. In medium bowl, beat ¾ cup sugar, the butter, egg and molasses with electric mixer on medium speed, or mix with spoon. Stir in flour, baking soda, cinnamon, ground ginger, cloves and salt. Cover and refrigerate at least 2 hours, until firm. 2. Heat oven to 350°F. Lightly spray cookie sheets with cooking spray. Place ¼ cup sugar in small bowl. Shape dough into ¾-inch balls; roll in sugar. Place balls about 2 inches apart on cookie sheet. Make indentation in center of each ball, using finger. Fill each indentation with slightly less than ¼ teaspoon of the marmalade. Sprinkle with crystallized ginger. 3. Bake 8 to 10 minutes or until set. Immediately transfer from cookie sheets to cooling racks. Cool completely, about 30 minutes.

Per Serving1 Cookie:

Calorie: 45 | fat: 1g | protein: 0g | carbs: 9g | sugars: 5g | fiber: 0g | sodium: 40mg

Simple Bread Pudding

Prep time: 25 minutes | Cook time: 40 minutes | Serves 8

6–8 slices bread, cubed
2 cups fat-free milk
2 eggs
¼ cup sugar
1 teaspoon ground cinnamon
1 teaspoon vanilla

1½ cups water
Sauce:
1 tablespoon cornstarch
6-ounce can concentrated grape juice

1. Place bread cubes in greased 1.6-quart baking dish. 2. Beat together milk and eggs. Stir in sugar, cinnamon and vanilla. Pour over bread and stir. 3. Cover with foil. 4. Place the trivet into your Instant Pot and pour in 1½ cup of water. Place a foil sling on top of the trivet, then place the baking dish on top. 5. Secure the lid and make sure lid is set to sealing. Press Manual and set time for 30 minutes. 6. When cook time is up, let the pressure release naturally for 15 minutes, then release any remaining pressure manually. Carefully remove the springform pan by using hot pads to lift the baking dish out by the foil sling. Let sit for a few minutes, uncovered, while you make the sauce. 7. Combine cornstarch and concentrated juice in saucepan. Heat until boiling, stirring constantly, until sauce is thickened. Serve drizzled over bread pudding.

Per Serving

Calories: 179 | fat: 2g | protein: 5g | carbs: 35g | sugars: 24g | fiber: 1g | sodium: 153mg

Crumb Pie Shell

Prep time: 10 minutes | Cook time: 10 minutes | Serves 10

1¼ cups finely crumbled high-fiber bran crisp breads (such as Fiber Rich+ Bran Crisp Breads)

2 tablespoons canola oil
1 tablespoon water
⅛ teaspoon cinnamon

1. Preheat the oven to 325 degrees. In a medium mixing bowl, combine all the ingredients, mixing thoroughly. 2. Spread the mixture evenly into a 10-inch pie pan. Press the mixture firmly onto the sides and bottom of the pan. 3. Bake the pie shell for 8–10 minutes. You can refrigerate it after baking until ready to use.

Per Serving

Calories: 78 | fat: 4g | protein: 2g | carbs: 10g | sugars: 1g | fiber: 1g | sodium: 99mg

Blueberry Chocolate Clusters

Prep time: 5 minutes | Cook time: 5 minutes | Serves 10

1½ cups dark chocolate chips
1 tablespoon coconut oil, melted

½ cups chopped, toasted pecans
2 cups blueberries

1. Line a baking sheet with parchment paper. 2. Melt the chocolate in a microwave-safe bowl in 20- to 30-second intervals. 3. In a medium bowl, combine the melted chocolate with the coconut oil and pecans. 4. Spoon a small amount of chocolate mixture (about 1 teaspoon) on the prepared baking sheet. 5. Place a cluster of about 5 blueberries on top of the chocolate. You should get about 20 clusters in total. 6. Drizzle a small amount of chocolate over the berries. 7. Freeze until set, about 15 minutes. 8. Store in an airtight container in the refrigerator for up to 5 days or in the freezer for up to 1 month.

Per Serving

Calories: 224 | fat: 17g | protein: 3g | carbs: 17g | sugars: 9g | fiber: 4g | sodium: 6mg

Chipotle Black Bean Brownies

Prep time: 15 minutes | Cook time: 30 minutes | Serves 8

Nonstick cooking spray
½ cup dark chocolate chips, divided
¾ cup cooked calypso beans or black beans
½ cup extra-virgin olive oil
2 large eggs
¼ cup unsweetened dark chocolate cocoa powder

⅓ cup honey
1 teaspoon vanilla extract
⅓ cup white wheat flour
½ teaspoon chipotle chili powder
½ teaspoon ground cinnamon
½ teaspoon baking powder
½ teaspoon kosher salt

1. Spray a 7-inch Bundt pan with nonstick cooking spray. 2. Place half of the chocolate chips in a small bowl and microwave them for 30 seconds. Stir and repeat, if necessary, until the chips have completely melted. 3. In a food processor, blend the beans and oil together. Add the melted chocolate chips, eggs, cocoa powder, honey, and vanilla. Blend until the mixture is smooth. 4. In a large bowl, whisk together the flour, chili powder, cinnamon, baking powder, and salt. Pour the bean mixture from the food processor into the bowl and stir with a wooden spoon until well combined. Stir in the remaining chocolate chips. 5. Pour the batter into the prepared Bundt pan. Cover loosely with foil. 6. Pour 1 cup of water into the electric pressure cooker. 7. Place the Bundt pan onto the wire rack and lower it into the pressure cooker. 8. Close and lock the lid of the pressure cooker. Set the valve to sealing. 9. Cook on high pressure for 30 minutes. 10. When the cooking is complete, hit Cancel and quick release the pressure. 11. Once the pin drops, unlock and remove the lid. 12. Carefully transfer the pan to a cooling rack for about 10 minutes, then invert the cake onto the rack and let it cool completely. 13. Cut into slices and serve.

Per Serving (1 slice):

Calories: 296 | fat: 20g | protein: 5g | carbs: 29g | sugars: 16g | fiber: 4g | sodium: 224mg

Baked Berry Cups with Crispy Cinnamon Wedges

Prep time: 25 minutes | Cook time: 30 minutes | Serves 4

2 teaspoons sugar
¾ teaspoon ground cinnamon
Butter-flavor cooking spray
1 balanced carb whole wheat tortilla (6 inch)
¼ cup sugar
2 tablespoons white whole wheat flour

1 teaspoon grated orange peel, if desired
1½ cups fresh blueberries
1½ cups fresh raspberries
About 1 cup fat-free whipped cream topping (from aerosol can)

1. Heat oven to 375°F. In sandwich-size resealable food-storage plastic bag, combine 2 teaspoons sugar and ½ teaspoon of the cinnamon. Using cooking spray, spray both sides of tortilla, about 3 seconds per side; cut tortilla into 8 wedges. In bag with cinnamon-sugar, add wedges; seal bag. Shake to coat wedges evenly. 2. On ungreased cookie sheet, spread out wedges. Bake 7 to 9 minutes, turning once, until just beginning to crisp (wedges will continue to crisp while cooling). Cool about 15 minutes. 3. Meanwhile, spray 4 (6-ounce) custard cups or ramekins with cooking spray; place cups on another cookie sheet. In small bowl, stir ¼ cup sugar, the flour, orange peel and remaining ¼ teaspoon cinnamon until blended. In medium bowl, gently toss berries with sugar mixture; divide evenly among custard cups. 4. Bake 15 minutes; stir gently. Bake 5 to 7 minutes longer or until liquid is bubbling around edges. Cool at least 15 minutes. 5. To serve, top each cup with about ¼ cup whipped cream topping; serve tortilla wedges with berry cups. Serve warm.

Per Serving

Calorie: 180 | fat: 2g | protein: 3g | carbs: 37g | sugars: 25g | fiber: 7g | sodium: 60mg

Chapter 9 Stews and Soups

Green Ginger Soup   90

Tasty Tomato Soup   90

Freshened-Up French Onion Soup   90

Chock-Full-of-Vegetables Chicken Soup   90

Coconut, Miso, and Sweet Potato White Bean
Chili   91

Chicken Noodle Soup   91

Turkey and Pinto Chili   91

Ham and Potato Chowder   92

Cauli-Curry Bean Soup   92

Unstuffed Cabbage Soup   92

Favorite Chili   92

Pumpkin Soup   93

French Onion Soup   93

Hearty Italian Minestrone   93

Four-Bean Field Stew   93

Comforting Chicken and Mushroom Soup   93

Black Bean, Turmeric, and Cauliflower Tortilla
Soup   94

Carrot Soup   94

Thai Peanut, Carrot, and Shrimp Soup   94

African Peanut Stew   94

Savory Beef Stew with Mushrooms and
Turnips   95

Butternut Squash Soup   95

Tomato and Kale Soup   95

French Market Soup   95

Egg Drop Soup   96

Southwestern Bean Soup with Corn
Dumplings   96

Potlikker Soup   96

Roasted Tomato and Sweet Potato Soup   96

Cauliflower Chili   97

Mexican Tortilla Soup   97

Instantly Good Beef Stew   97

Hearty Beef and Veggie Stew   97

Taco Soup   98

Chicken Brunswick Stew   98

Creamy Chicken Wild Rice Soup   98

Spicy Turkey Chili   98

Lentil Soup   99

Slow Cooker Chicken and Vegetable Soup   99

West African–Inspired Peanut Soup   99

Green Ginger Soup

Prep time: 10 minutes | Cook time: 30 minutes | Serves 2

½ cup chopped onion
½ cup peeled, chopped fennel
1 small zucchini, chopped
½ cup frozen lima beans
¼ cup uncooked brown rice
1 bay leaf
1 teaspoon dried basil
⅛ teaspoon freshly ground black pepper
2 cups water

1 cup frozen green beans
¼ cup fresh parsley, chopped
1 (3-inch) piece fresh ginger, peeled, grated, and pressed through a strainer to extract the juice (about 2 to 3 tablespoons)
Salt, to season
2 tablespoons chopped fresh chives

1. In a large pot set over medium-high heat, stir together the onion, fennel, zucchini, lima beans, rice, bay leaf, basil, pepper, and water. Bring to a boil. Reduce the heat to low. Simmer for 15 minutes. 2. Add the green beans. Simmer for about 5 minutes, uncovered, until tender. 3. Stir in the parsley. 4. Remove and discard the bay leaf. 5. In a blender or food processor, purée the soup in batches until smooth, adding water if necessary to thin. 6. Blend in the ginger juice. 7. Season with salt. Garnish with the chives. 8. Serve hot and enjoy immediately!

Per Serving

Calories: 189 | fat: 1.52g | protein: 7.14g | carbs: 38.58g | sugars: 3.1g | fiber: 6.8g | sodium: 338mg

Tasty Tomato Soup

Prep time: 10 minutes | Cook time: 1 hour 25 minutes | Serves 2

3 cups chopped tomatoes
1 red bell pepper, cut into chunks
2 tablespoons extra-virgin olive oil, divided
Salt, to season
Freshly ground black pepper, to season

1 medium onion, chopped
1 garlic clove, minced
2 cups low-sodium vegetable broth
1 cup sliced fresh button mushrooms
½ cup fresh chopped basil

1. Preheat the oven to 400°F. 2. On a baking sheet, spread out the tomatoes and red bell pepper. 3. Drizzle with 1 tablespoon of olive oil. Toss to coat. Season with salt and pepper. Place the sheet in the preheated oven. Roast for 45 minutes. 4. In a large stockpot set over medium heat, heat the remaining 1 tablespoon of olive oil. 5. Add the onion. Cook for 2 to 3 minutes, or until tender. 6. Stir in the garlic. Cook for 2 minutes more. 7. Add the vegetable broth, mushrooms, and basil. 8. Stir in the roasted tomatoes and peppers. Reduce the heat to medium-low. Cook for 30 minutes. 9. To a blender or food processor, carefully transfer the soup in batches, blending until smooth. Return the processed soup to the pot. Simmer for 5 minutes. 10. Serve warm and enjoy!

Per Serving

Calories: 255 | fat: 15.09g | protein: 5.97g | carbs: 28.64g | sugars: 17.95g | fiber: 6.6g | sodium: 738mg

Freshened-Up French Onion Soup

Prep time: 15 minutes | Cook time: 30 minutes | Serves 2

1 tablespoon extra-virgin olive oil
2 medium onions, sliced
2 cups low-sodium beef broth
1 (8-ounce) can chickpeas, drained and rinsed

½ teaspoon dried thyme
Salt
Freshly ground black pepper
4 slices nonfat Swiss deli-style cheese

1. In a medium soup pot set over medium-low heat, heat the olive oil. 2. Add the onions. Stir to coat them in oil. Cook for about 10 minutes, or until golden brown. 3. Add the beef broth, chickpeas, and thyme. Bring to a simmer. 4. Taste the broth. Season with salt and pepper. Cook for 10 minutes more. 5. Preheat the broiler to high. 6. Ladle the soup into 2 ovenproof soup bowls. 7. Top each with 2 slices of Swiss cheese. Place the bowls on a baking sheet. Carefully transfer the sheet to the preheated oven. Melt the cheese under the broiler for 2 minutes. Alternately, you can melt the cheese in the microwave (in microwave-safe bowls) on high in 30-second intervals until melted. 8. Enjoy immediately.

Per Serving

Calories: 278 | fat: 13.52g | protein: 15.39g | carbs: 28.6g | sugars: 3.04g | fiber: 1.8g | sodium: 804mg

Chock-Full-of-Vegetables Chicken Soup

Prep time: 5 minutes | Cook time: 15 minutes | Serves 2

1 tablespoon extra-virgin olive oil
8 ounces chicken tenders, cut into bite-size chunks
1 small zucchini, finely diced
1 cup sliced fresh button mushrooms
2 medium carrots, thinly sliced
2 celery stalks, thinly sliced

1 large shallot, finely chopped
1 garlic clove, minced
1 tablespoon dried parsley
1 teaspoon dried marjoram
⅛ teaspoon salt
2 plum tomatoes, chopped
2 cups reduced-sodium chicken broth
1½ cups packed baby spinach

1. In a large saucepan set over medium-high heat, heat olive oil. 2. Add the chicken. Cook for 3 to 4 minutes, stirring occasionally, or until browned. Transfer to a plate. Set aside. 3. To the saucepan, add the zucchini, mushrooms, carrots, celery, shallot, garlic, parsley, marjoram, and salt. Cook for 2 to 3 minutes, stirring frequently, until the vegetables are slightly softened. 4. Add the tomatoes and chicken broth. Increase the heat to high. Bring to a boil, stirring occasionally. Reduce the heat to low. Simmer for 5 minutes, or until the vegetables are tender. 5. Stir in the spinach, cooked chicken, and any accumulated juices on the plate. Cook for about 2 minutes, stirring, until the chicken is heated through. 6. Serve hot and enjoy!

Per Serving

Calories: 262 | fat: 9.56g | protein: 31.94g | carbs: 15.57g | sugars: 2.58g | fiber: 6.2g | sodium: 890mg

Coconut, Miso, and Sweet Potato White Bean Chili

Prep time: 10 minutes | Cook time: 35 minutes | Serves 4

2 teaspoons (10 ml) sesame oil, divided
1 medium white onion, coarsely chopped
2 teaspoons (6 g) minced fresh garlic
2 teaspoons (4 g) grated fresh ginger
1 tablespoon (17 g) miso of choice dissolved in 3 tablespoons (45 ml) warm water (see Tips)
1 (14-ounce [397-ml]) can light coconut milk
2 cups (480 ml) water

2 medium sweet potatoes, cubed
1 (15-ounce [425-g]) can navy beans, drained and rinsed
8 ounce (227 g) tempeh, crumbled (see Tips)
2 green onions, finely chopped
2 tablespoons (30 ml) low-sodium tamari
3 cups (200 g) coarsely chopped kale
Pinch of cayenne pepper (optional)
Sea salt, as needed
Black pepper, as needed

1. Heat 1 teaspoon of the oil in a large pot over medium heat. Add the onion, garlic, and ginger and sauté the mixture for about 5 minutes, or until the edges of the onion start to caramelize. 2. Add the miso-water mixture, coconut milk, water, sweet potatoes, and beans to the pot. Cover the pot and simmer the chili for about 30 minutes, or until the sweet potatoes are fork-tender. 3. Meanwhile, heat the remaining 1 teaspoon of oil in a medium skillet over medium heat. Add the tempeh, green onions, and tamari. Cook the mixture for 7 to 10 minutes, or until the tempeh is crispy. 4. Stir the tempeh mixture, kale, cayenne pepper (if using), sea salt, and black pepper into the chili, then serve.

Per Serving

Calorie: 407 | fat: 16g | protein: 22g | carbs: 45g | sugars: 5g | fiber: 12g | sodium: 1134mg

Chicken Noodle Soup

Prep time: 15 minutes | Cook time: 20 minutes | Serves 12

2 tablespoons avocado oil
1 medium onion, chopped
3 celery stalks, chopped
1 teaspoon kosher salt
¼ teaspoon freshly ground black pepper
2 teaspoons minced garlic
5 large carrots, peeled and cut into ¼-inch-thick rounds

3 pounds bone-in chicken breasts (about 3)
4 cups Chicken Bone Broth or low-sodium store-bought chicken broth
4 cups water
2 tablespoons soy sauce
6 ounces whole grain wide egg noodles

1. Set the electric pressure cooker to the Sauté setting. When the pot is hot, pour in the avocado oil. 2. Sauté the onion, celery, salt, and pepper for 3 to 5 minutes or until the vegetables begin to soften. 3. Add the garlic and carrots, and stir to mix well. Hit Cancel. 4. Add the chicken to the pot, meat-side down. Add the broth, water, and soy sauce. Close and lock the lid of the pressure cooker. Set the valve to sealing. 5. Cook on high pressure for 20 minutes. 6. When the cooking is complete, hit Cancel and quick release the pressure. Unlock and remove the lid. 7. Using tongs,

remove the chicken breasts to a cutting board. Hit Sauté/More and bring the soup to a boil. 8. Add the noodles and cook for 4 to 5 minutes or until the noodles are al dente. 9. While the noodles are cooking, use two forks to shred the chicken. Add the meat back to the pot and save the bones to make more bone broth. 10. Season with additional pepper, if desired, and serve.

Per Serving

Calories: 294 | fat: 13.92g | protein: 26.68g | carbs: 15.28g | sugars: 2.8g | fiber: 2.7g | sodium: 640mg

Turkey and Pinto Chili

Prep time: 0 minutes | Cook time: 60 minutes | Serves 8

2 tablespoons cold-pressed avocado oil
4 garlic cloves, diced
1 large yellow onion, diced
4 jalapeño chiles, seeded and diced
2 carrots, diced
4 celery stalks, diced
2 teaspoons fine sea salt
2 pounds 93 percent lean ground turkey
Two 4-ounce cans fire-roasted diced green chiles
4 tablespoons chili powder

2 teaspoons ground cumin
2 teaspoons ground coriander
1 teaspoon dried oregano
1 teaspoon dried sage
1 cup low-sodium chicken broth
3 cups drained cooked pinto beans, or two 15-ounce cans pinto beans, drained and rinsed
Two 14½-ounce cans no-salt petite diced tomatoes and their liquid
¼ cup tomato paste

1. Select the Sauté setting on the Instant Pot and heat the oil and garlic for 3 minutes, until the garlic is bubbling but not browned. Add the onion, jalapeños, carrots, celery, and salt and sauté for 5 minutes, until the onion begins to soften. Add the turkey and sauté, using a wooden spoon or spatula to break up the meat as it cooks, for 6 minutes, until cooked through and no streaks of pink remain. Stir in the green chiles, chili powder, cumin, coriander, oregano, sage, and broth, using a wooden spoon or spatula to nudge any browned bits from the bottom of the pot. 2. Pour in the beans in a layer on top of the turkey. Pour in the tomatoes and their liquid and add the tomato paste in a dollop on top. Do not stir in the beans, tomatoes, or tomato paste. 3. Secure the lid and set the Pressure Release to Sealing. Press the Cancel button to reset the cooking program, then select the Pressure Cook or Manual setting and set the cooking time for 15 minutes at high pressure. (The pot will take about 15 minutes to come up to pressure before the cooking program begins.) 4. When the cooking program ends, let the pressure release naturally for at least 20 minutes, then move the Pressure Release to Venting to release any remaining steam. Open the pot and stir the chili to mix all of the ingredients. 5. Press the Cancel button to reset the cooking program, then select the Sauté setting and set the cooking time for 10 minutes. Allow the chili to reduce and thicken. Do not stir the chili while it is cooking, as this will cause it to sputter more. 6. When the cooking program ends, the pot will turn off. Wearing heat-resistant mitts, remove the inner pot from the housing. Wait for about 2 minutes to allow the chili to stop simmering, then give it a final stir. 7. Ladle the chili into bowls and serve hot.

Per Serving

Calories: 354 | fat: 14g | protein: 30g | carbs: 28g | sugars: 6g | fiber: 9g | sodium: 819mg

Chapter 9 Stews and Soups | 91

Ham and Potato Chowder

Prep time: 25 minutes | Cook time: 8 hour s | Serves 5

5-ounce package scalloped potatoes
Sauce mix from potato package
1 cup extra-lean, reduced-sodium, cooked ham, cut into narrow strips
4 teaspoons sodium-free bouillon powder
4 cups water
1 cup chopped celery
⅓ cup chopped onions
Pepper to taste
2 cups fat-free half-and-half
⅓ cup flour

1. Combine potatoes, sauce mix, ham, bouillon powder, water, celery, onions, and pepper in the inner pot of the Instant Pot. 2. Secure the lid and cook using the Slow Cook function on low for 7 hours. 3. Combine half-and-half and flour. Remove the lid and gradually add to the inner pot, blending well. 4. Secure the lid once more and cook on the low Slow Cook function for up to 1 hour more, stirring occasionally until thickened.

Per Serving

Calories: 241 | fat: 3g | protein: 11g | carbs: 41g | sugars: 8g | fiber: 3g | sodium: 836mg

Cauli-Curry Bean Soup

Prep time: 10 minutes | Cook time: 25 minutes | Serves 8

2 cups chopped onion
1½ cups chopped carrot or sweet potato
1½ tablespoons curry powder (or to taste; use more if you really love curry)
1¼ teaspoons sea salt
Freshly ground black pepper to taste
1 teaspoon mustard seeds
1 teaspoon ground cumin
1 teaspoon ground turmeric
¼ teaspoon ground cardamom
⅛ teaspoon ground cinnamon
4–5 tablespoons + 4 cups water
3–4 cups cauliflower florets
1 can (15 ounces) chickpeas, rinsed and drained
1 can (15 ounces) adzuki or black beans, rinsed and drained
1 cup dried red lentils
1 can (28 ounces) crushed tomatoes
1 tablespoon grated fresh ginger
1–2 teaspoons pure maple syrup (optional)

1. In a large pot over medium-high heat, combine the onion, carrot or sweet potato, curry powder, salt, pepper, mustard seeds, cumin, turmeric, cardamom, cinnamon, and 3 tablespoons of the water. Stir, cover, and cook for 4 to 5 minutes, stirring occasionally. (Add another 1 to 2 tablespoons of water if needed to keep the vegetables and spices from sticking.) Add the cauliflower, chickpeas, beans, lentils, tomatoes, and remaining 4 cups water. Stir and increase the heat to high to bring to a boil. Reduce the heat to low, cover, and simmer for 15 to 20 minutes. Stir in the ginger and syrup (if using). Season to taste, and serve.

Per Serving

Calorie: 226 | fat: 2g | protein: 14g | carbs: 42g | sugars: 7g | fiber: 13g | sodium: 577mg

Unstuffed Cabbage Soup

Prep time: 15 minutes | Cook time: 20 minutes | Serves 5

2 tablespoons coconut oil
1 pound ground sirloin or turkey
1 medium onion, diced
2 cloves garlic, minced
1 small head cabbage, chopped, cored, cut into roughly 2-inch pieces.
6-ounce can low-sodium tomato paste
32-ounce can low-sodium diced tomatoes, with liquid
2 cups low-sodium beef broth
1½ cups water
¾ cup brown rice
1–2 teaspoons salt
½ teaspoon black pepper
1 teaspoon oregano
1 teaspoon parsley

1. Melt coconut oil in the inner pot of the Instant Pot using Sauté function. Add ground meat. Stir frequently until meat loses color, about 2 minutes. 2. Add onion and garlic and continue to sauté for 2 more minutes, stirring frequently. 3. Add chopped cabbage. 4. On top of cabbage layer tomato paste, tomatoes with liquid, beef broth, water, rice, and spices. 5. Secure the lid and set vent to sealing. Using Manual setting, select 20 minutes. 6. When time is up, let the pressure release naturally for 10 minutes, then do a quick release.

Per Serving

Calories: 282 | fat: 6g | protein: 23g | carbs: 34g | sugars: 6g | fiber: 3g | sodium: 898mg

Favorite Chili

Prep time: 10 minutes | Cook time: 35 minutes | Serves 5

1 pound extra-lean ground beef
1 teaspoon salt
½ teaspoons black pepper
1 tablespoon olive oil
1 small onion, chopped
2 cloves garlic, minced
1 green pepper, chopped
2 tablespoons chili powder
½ teaspoons cumin
1 cup water
16-ounce can chili beans
15-ounce can low-sodium crushed tomatoes

1. Press Sauté button and adjust once to Sauté More function. Wait until indicator says "hot." 2. Season the ground beef with salt and black pepper. 3. Add the olive oil into the inner pot. Coat the whole bottom of the pot with the oil. 4. Add ground beef into the inner pot. The ground beef will start to release moisture. Allow the ground beef to brown and crisp slightly, stirring occasionally to break it up. Taste and adjust the seasoning with more salt and ground black pepper. 5. Add diced onion, minced garlic, chopped pepper, chili powder, and cumin. Sauté for about 5 minutes, until the spices start to release their fragrance. Stir frequently. 6. Add water and 1 can of chili beans, not drained. Mix well. Pour in 1 can of crushed tomatoes. 7. Close and secure lid, making sure vent is set to sealing, and pressure cook on Manual at high pressure for 10 minutes. 8. Let the pressure release naturally when cooking time is up. Open the lid carefully.

Per Serving

Calories: 213 | fat: 10g | protein: 18g | carbs: 11g | sugars: 4g | fiber: 4g | sodium: 385mg

Pumpkin Soup

Prep time: 15 minutes | Cook time: 30 minutes | Serves 6

2 cups store-bought low-sodium seafood broth, divided
1 bunch collard greens, stemmed and cut into ribbons
1 tomato, chopped
1 garlic clove, minced
1 butternut squash or other

winter squash, peeled and cut into 1-inch cubes
1 teaspoon paprika
1 teaspoon dried dill
2 (5-ounce) cans boneless, skinless salmon in water, rinsed

1. In a heavy-bottomed large stockpot, bring ½ cup of broth to a simmer over medium heat. 2. Add the collard greens, tomato, and garlic and cook for 5 minutes, or until the greens are wilted and the garlic is softened. 3. Add the squash, paprika, dill, and remaining 1½ cups of broth. Cover and cook for 20 minutes, or until the squash is tender. 4. Add the salmon and cook for 3 minutes, or just enough for the flavors to come together.

Per Serving

Calories: 161 | fat: 5.5g | protein: 23.92g | carbs: 4.51g | sugars: 1.18g | fiber: 1g | sodium: 579mg

French Onion Soup

Prep time: 10 minutes | Cook time: 20 minutes | Serves 10

½ cup light, soft tub margarine
8–10 large onions, sliced
3 14-ounce cans 98% fat-free, lower-sodium beef broth
2½ cups water
3 teaspoons sodium-free

chicken bouillon powder
1½ teaspoons Worcestershire sauce
3 bay leaves
10 (1-ounce) slices French bread, toasted

1. Turn the Instant Pot to the Sauté function and add in the margarine and onions. Cook about 5 minutes, or until the onions are slightly soft. Press Cancel. 2. Add the beef broth, water, bouillon powder, Worcestershire sauce, and bay leaves and stir. 3. Secure the lid and make sure vent is set to sealing. Cook on Manual mode for 20 minutes. 4. Let the pressure release naturally for 15 minutes, then do a quick release. Open the lid and discard bay leaves. 5. Ladle into bowls. Top each with a slice of bread and some cheese if you desire.

Per Serving

Calories: 178 | fat: 4g | protein: 6g | carbs: 31g | sugars: 10g | fiber: 4g | sodium: 476mg

Hearty Italian Minestrone

Prep time: 10 minutes | Cook time: 50 minutes | Serves 8

½ cup sliced onion
1 tablespoon extra-virgin olive oil
4 cups low-sodium chicken broth
¾ cup diced carrot
½ cup diced potato (with skin)
2 cups sliced cabbage or

coarsely chopped spinach
1 cup diced zucchini
½ cup cooked garbanzo beans (drained and rinsed, if canned)
½ cup cooked navy beans (drained and rinsed, if canned)
One 14.5-ounce can low-sodium tomatoes, with liquid

½ cup diced celery
2 tablespoons fresh basil, finely chopped
½ cup uncooked whole-wheat

rotini or other shaped pasta
2 tablespoons fresh parsley, finely chopped, for garnish

1. In a large stockpot over medium heat, sauté the onion in oil until the onion is slightly browned. Add the chicken broth, carrot, and potato. Cover and cook over medium heat for 30 minutes. 2. Add the remaining ingredients and cook for an additional 15–20 minutes, until the pasta is cooked through. Garnish with parsley and serve hot.

Per Serving

Calories: 101 | fat: 2.01g | protein: 5.86g | carbs: 16.51g | sugars: 4.45g | fiber: 3.9g | sodium: 108mg

Four-Bean Field Stew

Prep time: 10 minutes | Cook time: 40 minutes | Serves 8 to 10

6 cups store-bought low-sodium vegetable broth
1 cup dried lima beans
1 cup dried black beans
1 cup dried pinto beans
1 cup dried kidney beans
1 cup roughly chopped tomato
2 carrots, peeled and roughly chopped

1 zucchini, chopped
½ cup chopped white onion
1 celery stalk, roughly chopped
2 garlic cloves, minced
1 teaspoon dried oregano
1 teaspoon dried thyme
¼ teaspoon freshly ground black pepper

1. In an electric pressure cooker, combine the broth, lima beans, black beans, pinto beans, kidney beans, tomato, carrots, zucchini, onion, celery, garlic, oregano, thyme, and pepper. 2. Close and lock the lid, and set the pressure valve to sealing. 3. Select the Manual/Pressure Cook setting, and cook for 40 minutes. 4. Once cooking is complete, quick-release the pressure. Carefully remove the lid. 5. Serve.

Per Serving

Calories: 262 | fat: 2.98g | protein: 14.57g | carbs: 46.7g | sugars: 7.74g | fiber: 10.4g | sodium: 143mg

Comforting Chicken and Mushroom Soup

Prep time: 5 minutes | Cook time: 20 minutes | Serves 6

1 quart low-sodium chicken broth
1 tablespoon light soy sauce
1 cup sliced mushrooms, stems removed

1 tablespoon finely chopped scallions
1 tablespoon dry sherry
½ pound boneless, skinless chicken breast, cubed

1. In a stockpot, simmer all ingredients except the chicken for 10 minutes. 2. Add the chicken cubes, and simmer for 6–8 minutes more. Serve with additional soy sauce if desired (but be aware that this will raise the sodium level of the soup).

Per Serving

Calories: 88 | fat: 4.44g | protein: 9.64g | carbs: 2.27g | sugars: 1.17g | fiber: 0.2g | sodium: 88mg

Black Bean, Turmeric, and Cauliflower Tortilla Soup

Prep time: 10 minutes | Cook time: 45 minutes | Serves 4

1 medium head cauliflower, chopped into medium florets
2 teaspoons (10 ml) extra virgin olive oil, divided
½ teaspoons ground turmeric
½ teaspoons garlic powder
1 medium yellow onion, coarsely chopped
1 clove garlic, minced
1 medium red bell pepper, coarsely chopped
2 cups (480 ml) low-sodium salsa
1 teaspoon chipotle chili powder (see Tips)
4 cups (960 ml) water
Juice of ½ medium lime
1 (15-ounce [425-g]) can black beans, drained and rinsed
½ cup (60 g) shredded Cheddar cheese
Finely chopped fresh cilantro, as needed
Avocado, sliced (optional)
4 lime wedges

1. Preheat the oven to 425°F (218°C). 2. Place the cauliflower florets in a large bowl. Add 1 teaspoon of the oil, turmeric, and garlic powder and toss the cauliflower florets to coat them in the seasonings. Transfer the cauliflower to a large baking sheet. Bake the cauliflower for 25 minutes, until it is golden brown. 3. Meanwhile, heat the remaining 1 teaspoon of oil in a large pot over medium heat. Add the onion, garlic, and bell pepper and sauté the vegetables for 5 to 10 minutes, or until the onion is translucent with charred edges. Add the salsa, chipotle chili powder, water, lime juice, and black beans and bring the soup to a simmer. 4. When the cauliflower is done, add it and the Cheddar cheese to the soup. Simmer the soup for at least 15 to 20 minutes to allow the flavors to meld. 5. Serve the soup with the cilantro sprinkled on top, avocado if desired, and a lime wedge on the side of each serving.

Per Serving

Calorie: 347 | fat: 7g | protein: 13g | carbs: 62g | sugars: 15g | fiber: 13g | sodium: 268mg

Carrot Soup

Prep time: 15 minutes | Cook time: 25 minutes | Serves 6

4 cups store-bought low-sodium vegetable broth, divided
2 celery stalks, halved
1 small yellow onion, roughly chopped
½ fennel bupounds, cored and roughly chopped
1 (1-inch) piece fresh ginger, peeled and chopped
1 pound carrots, peeled and halved
2 teaspoons ground cumin
1 garlic clove, peeled
1 tablespoon almond butter

1. Select the Sauté setting on an electric pressure cooker, and combine ½ cup of broth, the celery, onion, fennel, and ginger. Cook for 5 minutes, or until the vegetables are tender. 2. Add the carrots, cumin, garlic, remaining 3½ cups of broth, and the almond butter. 3. Close and lock the lid, and set the pressure valve to sealing. 4. Change to the Manual/Pressure Cook setting, and cook for 15 minutes. 5. Once cooking is complete, quick-release the pressure. Carefully remove the lid, and let cool for 5 minutes. 6. Using a stand mixer or an immersion blender,

carefully purée the soup. Serve with a heaping plate of greens.

Per Serving

Calories: 97 | fat: 2.88g | protein: 2.86g | carbs: 17.21g | sugars: 9.73g | fiber: 4g | sodium: 177mg

Thai Peanut, Carrot, and Shrimp Soup

Prep time: 10 minutes | Cook time: 10 minutes | Serves 4

1 tablespoon coconut oil
1 tablespoon Thai red curry paste
½ onion, sliced
3 garlic cloves, minced
2 cups chopped carrots
½ cup whole unsalted peanuts
4 cups low-sodium vegetable broth
½ cup unsweetened plain almond milk
½ pound shrimp, peeled and deveined
Minced fresh cilantro, for garnish

1. In a large pan, heat the oil over medium-high heat until shimmering. 2. Add the curry paste and cook, stirring constantly, for 1 minute. Add the onion, garlic, carrots, and peanuts to the pan, and continue to cook for 2 to 3 minutes until the onion begins to soften. 3. Add the broth and bring to a boil. Reduce the heat to low and simmer for 5 to 6 minutes until the carrots are tender. 4. Using an immersion blender or in a blender, purée the soup until smooth and return it to the pot. With the heat still on low, add the almond milk and stir to combine. Add the shrimp to the pot and cook for 2 to 3 minutes until cooked through. 5. Garnish with cilantro and serve.

Per Serving

Calories: 237 | fat: 14g | protein: 14g | carbs: 17g | sugars: 6g | fiber: 5g | sodium: 619mg

African Peanut Stew

Prep time: 10 minutes | Cook time: 35 minutes | Serves 2

3 cups low-sodium vegetable broth
1 small onion, chopped
1 small red bell pepper, chopped
1 medium carrot, chopped
1 tablespoon minced fresh ginger
2 garlic cloves, minced
¼ teaspoon salt, plus more to season
½ cup unsalted natural peanut butter
2 tablespoons tomato paste
1 bunch kale, thoroughly washed, deveined, and chopped (about 2½ cups)
Freshly ground black pepper, to season
2 scallions, chopped

1. In a medium pot set over medium-low heat, bring the vegetable broth to a boil. 2. Add the onion, bell pepper, carrot, ginger, garlic, and salt. Cook for 20 minutes. 3. In a medium, heat-safe mixing bowl, stir together the peanut butter and tomato paste. 4. Transfer 1 cup of the hot vegetable broth to the bowl. Whisk until smooth. Pour the peanut butter mixture back into the soup. Mix well to combine. 5. Stir in the kale. Season with salt and pepper. Simmer for about 15 minutes more, stirring frequently. 6. Top with the scallions and enjoy!

Per Serving

Calories: 565 | fat: 35.52g | protein: 23.74g | carbs: 49g | sugars: 26.24g | fiber: 11.8g | sodium: 580mg

Savory Beef Stew with Mushrooms and Turnips

Prep time: 0 minutes | Cook time: 55 minutes | Serves 6

1½ pounds beef stew meat
¾ teaspoon fine sea salt
¾ teaspoon freshly ground black pepper
1 tablespoon cold-pressed avocado oil
3 garlic cloves, minced
1 yellow onion, diced
2 celery stalks, diced
8 ounces cremini mushrooms, quartered
1 cup low-sodium roasted beef bone broth
2 tablespoons Worcestershire

sauce
1 tablespoon Dijon mustard
1 teaspoon dried rosemary, crumbled
1 bay leaf
3 tablespoons tomato paste
8 ounces carrots, cut into 1-inch-thick rounds
1 pound turnips, cut into 1-inch pieces
1 pound parsnips, halved lengthwise, then cut crosswise into 1-inch pieces

1. Sprinkle the beef all over with the salt and pepper. 2. Select the Sauté setting on the Instant Pot and heat the oil and garlic for 2 minutes, until the garlic is bubbling but not browned. Add the onion, celery, and mushrooms and sauté for 5 minutes, until the onion begins to soften and the mushrooms are giving up their liquid. Stir in the broth, Worcestershire sauce, mustard, rosemary, and bay leaf. Stir in the beef. Add the tomato paste in a dollop on top. Do not stir it in. 3. Secure the lid and set the Pressure Release to Sealing. Press the Cancel button to reset the cooking program, then select the Meat/Stew, Pressure Cook, or Manual setting and set the cooking time for 20 minutes at high pressure. (The pot will take about 10 minutes to come up to pressure before the cooking program begins.) 4. When the cooking program ends, perform a quick pressure release by moving the Pressure Release to Venting, or let the pressure release naturally. Open the pot, remove and discard the bay leaf, and stir in the tomato paste. Place the carrots, turnips, and parsnips on top of the meat. 5. Secure the lid and set the Pressure Release to Sealing. Press the Cancel button to reset the cooking program, then select the Pressure Cook or Manual setting and set the cooking time for 3 minutes at low pressure. (The pot will take about 15 minutes to come up to pressure before the cooking program begins.) 6. When the cooking program ends, perform a quick pressure release by moving the Pressure Release to Venting. Open the pot and stir to combine all of the ingredients. 7. Ladle the stew into bowls and serve hot.

Per Serving

Calories: 304 | fat: 8g | protein: 29g | carbs: 30g | sugars: 10g | fiber: 8g | sodium: 490mg

Butternut Squash Soup

Prep time: 30 minutes | Cook time: 15 minutes | Serves 4

2 tablespoons margarine
1 large onion, chopped
2 cloves garlic, minced
1 teaspoon thyme
½ teaspoon sage
Salt and pepper to taste

2 large butternut squash, peeled, seeded, and cubed (about 4 pounds)
4 cups low-sodium chicken stock

1. In the inner pot of the Instant Pot, melt the margarine using Sauté function. 2. Add onion and garlic and cook until soft, 3 to 5 minutes. 3. Add thyme and sage and cook another minute. Season with salt and pepper. 4. Stir in butternut squash and add chicken stock. 5. Secure the lid and make sure vent is at sealing. Using Manual setting, cook squash and seasonings 10 minutes, using high pressure. 6. When time is up, do a quick release of the pressure. 7. Puree the soup in a food processor or use immersion blender right in the inner pot. If soup is too thick, add more stock. Adjust salt and pepper as needed.

Per Serving

Calories: 279 | fat: 7g | protein: 6g | carbs: 48g | sugars: 10g | fiber: 9g | sodium: 144mg

Tomato and Kale Soup

Prep time: 10 minutes | Cook time: 15 minutes | Serves 4

1 tablespoon extra-virgin olive oil
1 medium onion, chopped
2 carrots, finely chopped
3 garlic cloves, minced
4 cups low-sodium vegetable broth

1 (28-ounce) can crushed tomatoes
½ teaspoon dried oregano
¼ teaspoon dried basil
4 cups chopped baby kale leaves
¼ teaspoon salt

1. In a large pot, heat the oil over medium heat. Add the onion and carrots to the pan. Sauté for 3 to 5 minutes until they begin to soften. Add the garlic and sauté for 30 seconds more, until fragrant. 2. Add the vegetable broth, tomatoes, oregano, and basil to the pot and bring to a boil. Reduce the heat to low and simmer for 5 minutes. 3. Using an immersion blender, purée the soup. 4. Add the kale and simmer for 3 more minutes. Season with the salt. Serve immediately.

Per Serving

Calories: 170 | fat: 5g | protein: 6g | carbs: 31g | sugars: 13g | fiber: 9g | sodium: 600mg

French Market Soup

Prep time: 20 minutes | Cook time: 1 hour | Serves 8

2 cups mixed dry beans, washed with stones removed
7 cups water
1 ham hock, all visible fat removed
1 teaspoon salt
¼ teaspoon pepper

16-ounce can low-sodium tomatoes
1 large onion, chopped
1 garlic clove, minced
1 chile, chopped, or 1 teaspoon chili powder
¼ cup lemon juice

1. Combine all ingredients in the inner pot of the Instant Pot. 2. Secure the lid and make sure vent is set to sealing. Using Manual, set the Instant Pot to cook for 60 minutes. 3. When cooking time is over, let the pressure release naturally. When the Instant Pot is ready, unlock the lid, then remove the bone and any hard or fatty pieces. Pull the meat off the bone and chop into small pieces. Add the ham back into the Instant Pot.

Per Serving

Calories: 191 | fat: 4g | protein: 12g | carbs: 29g | sugars: 5g | fiber: 7g | sodium: 488mg

Egg Drop Soup

Prep time: 10 minutes | Cook time: 15 minutes | Serves 4

3½ cups low-sodium vegetable broth, divided
1 teaspoon grated fresh ginger (optional)
2 garlic cloves, minced
3 teaspoons low-sodium soy

sauce or tamari
1 tablespoon cornstarch
2 large eggs, lightly beaten
2 scallions, both white and green parts, thinly sliced

1. In a large saucepan, bring 3 cups plus 6 tablespoons of vegetable broth and the ginger (if using), garlic, and tamari to a boil over medium-high heat. 2. In a small bowl, make a slurry by combining the cornstarch and the remaining 2 tablespoons of broth. Stir until dissolved. Slowly add the cornstarch mixture to the rest of the heated soup, stirring until thickened, 2 to 3 minutes. 3. Reduce the heat to low and simmer. While stirring the soup, pour the eggs in slowly. Turn off the heat, add the scallions, and serve. 4. Store the cooled soup in an airtight container in the refrigerator for up to 3 days.

Per Serving

Calories: 82 | fat: 2.99g | protein: 3.79g | carbs: 11.42g | sugars: 6.33g | fiber: 1.2g | sodium: 248mg

Southwestern Bean Soup with Corn Dumplings

Prep time: 50 minutes | Cook time: 4 to 12 hours | Serves 8

15½-ounce can red kidney beans, rinsed and drained
15½-ounce can black beans, pinto beans, or great northern beans, rinsed and drained
3 cups water
14½-ounce can Mexican-style stewed tomatoes
10-ounce package frozen whole-kernel corn, thawed
1 cup sliced carrots
1 cup chopped onions
4-ounce can chopped green chilies

3 teaspoons sodium-free instant bouillon powder (any flavor)
1–2 teaspoons chili powder
2 cloves garlic, minced
Sauce:
⅓ cup flour
¼ cup yellow cornmeal
1 teaspoon baking powder
Dash of pepper
1 egg white, beaten
2 tablespoons milk
1 tablespoon oil

1. Combine the 11 soup ingredients in inner pot of the Instant Pot. 2. Secure the lid and cook on the Low Slow Cook setting for 10–12 hours or high for 4–5 hours. 3. Make dumplings by mixing together flour, cornmeal, baking powder, and pepper. 4. Combine egg white, milk, and oil. Add to flour mixture. Stir with fork until just combined. 5. At the end of the soup's cooking time, turn the Instant Pot to Slow Cook function high if you don't already have it there. Remove the lid and drop dumpling mixture by rounded teaspoonfuls to make 8 mounds atop the soup. 6. Secure the lid once more and cook for an additional 30 minutes.

Per Serving

Calories: 197 | fat: 1g | protein: 9g | carbs: 39g | sugars: 6g | fiber: 8g | sodium: 367mg

Potlikker Soup

Prep time: 15 minutes | Cook time: 20 minutes | Serves 6

3 cups store-bought low-sodium chicken broth, divided
1 medium onion, chopped
3 garlic cloves, minced
1 bunch collard greens or mustard greens including stems, roughly chopped

1 fresh ham bone
5 carrots, peeled and cut into 1-inch rounds
2 fresh thyme sprigs
3 bay leaves
Freshly ground black pepper

1. Select the Sauté setting on an electric pressure cooker, and combine ½ cup of chicken broth, the onion, and garlic and cook for 3 to 5 minutes, or until the onion and garlic are translucent. 2. Add the collard greens, ham bone, carrots, remaining 2½ cups of broth, the thyme, and bay leaves. 3. Close and lock the lid and set the pressure valve to sealing. 4. Change to the Manual/Pressure Cook setting, and cook for 15 minutes. 5. Once cooking is complete, quick-release the pressure. Carefully remove the lid. Discard the bay leaves. 6. Serve.

Per Serving

Calories: 107 | fat: 2.61g | protein: 11.74g | carbs: 11.83g | sugars: 2.62g | fiber: 4.7g | sodium: 556mg

Roasted Tomato and Sweet Potato Soup

Prep time: 10 minutes | Cook time: 40 to 50 minutes | Serves 4

1½ cups onions, finely chopped
2 cups cubed red or yellow potatoes (not russet)
2 cups cubed sweet potatoes (can use frozen)
3–4 large cloves garlic, minced
1¼ teaspoons sea salt
1½ cups peeled, quartered onion (roughly 1 large onion)
4 cups cubed sweet potato (roughly 1–1¼ pounds before peeling)

4 cups (about 1½ pounds) quartered Roma or other tomatoes, juices squeezed out
1½ teaspoons dried basil
1½ teaspoons dried oregano
1 tablespoon balsamic vinegar
1 teaspoon blackstrap molasses
Freshly ground black pepper to taste
1⅛ teaspoons sea salt
2¼–2½ cups water
¼ cup chopped fresh basil (optional)

1. Preheat the oven to 450°F. 2. In a large baking dish, combine the onion, sweet potato, tomatoes, basil, oregano, vinegar, molasses, pepper, and 1 teaspoon of the salt. Cook for 40 to 50 minutes, stirring a couple of times, until the sweet potatoes are softened and the mixture is becoming caramelized. Transfer the vegetables and any juices they've released in the pan to a medium soup pot, add 2¼ cups of the water and the remaining ⅛ teaspoon salt, and use an immersion blender to puree. (Alternatively, you can transfer everything to a blender to puree.) Blend to the desired smoothness, using the additional ¼ cup water if needed. Stir in fresh basil, if using, and serve.

Per Serving

Calorie: 152 | fat: 0.4g | protein: 4g | carbs: 35g | sugars: 14g | fiber: 5g | sodium: 648mg

Cauliflower Chili

Prep time: 10 minutes | Cook time: 35 minutes | Serves 5

2 cups thickly sliced carrot
½ large or 1 full small head cauliflower
4 or 5 cloves garlic, minced
1 tablespoon balsamic vinegar
1½ cups diced onion
1 teaspoon sea salt
1½ tablespoons mild chili powder
1 tablespoon cocoa powder
2 teaspoons ground cumin
2 teaspoons dried oregano
⅛ teaspoon allspice
¼ teaspoon crushed red-pepper flakes (or to taste)
1 can (28 ounces) crushed tomatoes
1 can (15 ounces) pinto beans, rinsed and drained
1 can (15 ounces) kidney beans or black beans, rinsed and drained
½ cup water
Lime wedges

1. In a food processor, combine the carrot, cauliflower, and garlic, and pulse until finely minced. (Alternatively, you could mince by hand.) In a large pot over medium heat, combine the vinegar, onion, salt, chili powder, cocoa, cumin, oregano, allspice, and red-pepper flakes. Cook for 3 to 4 minutes, stirring occasionally. Add the minced carrot, cauliflower, and garlic, and cook for 5 to 6 minutes, stirring occasionally. Add the tomatoes, pinto and kidney beans, and water, and stir to combine. Increase the heat to high to bring to a boil. Reduce the heat to low, cover, and simmer for 25 minutes. Taste, and season as desired. Serve with lime wedges.

Per Serving

Calorie: 237 | fat: 3g | protein: 13g | carbs: 40g | sugars: 13g | fiber: 15g | sodium: 1036mg

Mexican Tortilla Soup

Prep time: 10 minutes | Cook time: 40 minutes | Serves 8

2 tablespoons extra-virgin olive oil
1 onion, chopped
2 cloves garlic, minced
¼ cup freshly chopped cilantro
1 tablespoon cumin
1 teaspoon cayenne pepper
1 quart low-sodium chicken broth
One 15-ounce can low-sodium
whole tomatoes, drained and coarsely chopped
1 medium zucchini, sliced
1 medium yellow squash, sliced
1 cup yellow corn
Six 6-inch corn tortillas
½ cup reduced-fat shredded cheddar cheese

1. Preheat the oven to 350 degrees. 2. In a large saucepan, heat the oil, and sauté the onion and garlic for 5 minutes. 3. Add the cilantro, cumin, and cayenne pepper; sauté for 3 more minutes. Add the remaining ingredients except the tortillas and cheese. Bring to a boil; cover and let simmer for 30 minutes. 4. Cut each tortilla into about 10 strips (use a pizza cutter to do this easily). Place the strips on a cookie sheet and bake for 5–6 minutes at 350 degrees until slightly browned and toasted. Remove from the oven. 5. To serve the soup, place strips of tortilla into each bowl. Ladle the soup on top of the tortilla strips. Top with cheese.

Per Serving

Calories: 193 | fat: 4.48g | protein: 9.22g | carbs: 31.23g | sugars: 3.25g | fiber: 3.4g | sodium: 172mg

Instantly Good Beef Stew

Prep time: 20 minutes | Cook time: 35 minutes | Serves 6

3 tablespoons olive oil, divided
2 pounds stewing beef, cubed
2 cloves garlic, minced
1 large onion, chopped
3 ribs celery, sliced
3 large potatoes, cubed
2–3 carrots, sliced
8 ounces no-salt-added tomato
sauce
10 ounces low-sodium beef broth
2 teaspoons Worcestershire sauce
¼ teaspoon pepper
1 bay leaf

1. Set the Instant Pot to the Sauté function, then add in 1 tablespoon of the oil. Add in ⅓ of the beef cubes and brown and sear all sides. Repeat this process twice more with the remaining oil and beef cubes. Set the beef aside. 2. Place the garlic, onion, and celery into the pot and sauté for a few minutes. Press Cancel. 3. Add the beef back in as well as all of the remaining ingredients. 4. Secure the lid and make sure the vent is set to sealing. Choose Manual for 35 minutes. 5. When cook time is up, let the pressure release naturally for 15 minutes, then release any remaining pressure manually. 6. Remove the lid, remove the bay leaf, then serve.

Per Serving

Calories: 401 | fat: 20g | protein: 35g | carbs: 19g | sugars: 5g | fiber: 3g | sodium: 157mg

Hearty Beef and Veggie Stew

Prep time: 15 minutes | Cook time: 45 minutes | Serves 4

2 tablespoons (30 ml) avocado oil
1 pound (454 g) extra lean beef stew meat
1 medium yellow onion, cut into large chunks
4 large carrots, cut into 2-inch (5-cm) chunks
5 to 6 small red potatoes,
quartered
3 cups (720 ml) low-sodium beef broth
½ teaspoons salt
½ teaspoons black pepper
¼ to ⅓ cup (16 to 21 g) finely chopped fresh herbs of choice (see Tip)

1. Heat the oil in a large Dutch oven or pot over medium-high heat. 2. Add the stew meat and cook it for 2 to 3 minutes on each side, until it is brown on all sides but still pink in the center. Remove the stew meat from the Dutch oven and set it aside. 3. Add the onion and carrots to the Dutch oven and cook them for 5 to 10 minutes, until they start to soften. 4. Add the potatoes, broth, salt, black pepper, and herbs. Bring the mixture to a boil. Reduce the heat to low and simmer the stew for 30 minutes, until the vegetables are fork-tender. 5. Add the stew meat to the stew and cook it for 5 to 10 minutes to warm the meat through. Serve the stew immediately.

Per Serving

Calorie: 400 | fat: 11g | protein: 32g | carbs: 45g | sugars: 8g | fiber: 6g | sodium: 742mg

Chapter 9 Stews and Soups | 97

Taco Soup

Prep time: 5 minutes | Cook time: 20 minutes | Serves 4

Avocado oil cooking spray	½ teaspoon chili powder
1 medium red bell pepper, chopped	½ teaspoon garlic powder
½ cup chopped yellow onion	2 cups low-sodium beef broth
1 pound 93% lean ground beef	1 (15-ounce) can no-salt-added diced tomatoes
1 teaspoon ground cumin	1½ cups frozen corn
½ teaspoon salt	⅓ cup half-and-half

1. Heat a large stockpot over medium-low heat. When hot, coat the cooking surface with cooking spray. Put the pepper and onion in the pan and cook for 5 minutes. 2. Add the ground beef, cumin, salt, chili powder, and garlic powder. Cook for 5 to 7 minutes, stirring and breaking apart the beef as needed. 3. Add the broth, diced tomatoes with their juices, and corn. Increase the heat to medium-high and simmer for 10 minutes. 4. Remove from the heat and stir in the half-and-half.

Per Serving

Calories: 487 | fat: 21.71g | protein: 39.49g | carbs: 34.67g | sugars: 8.43g | fiber: 4.8g | sodium: 437mg

Chicken Brunswick Stew

Prep time: 0 minutes | Cook time: 30 minutes | Serves 6

2 tablespoons extra-virgin olive oil	broth
2 garlic cloves, chopped	1 tablespoon hot sauce (such as Tabasco or Crystal)
1 large yellow onion, diced	1 tablespoon raw apple cider vinegar
2 pounds boneless, skinless chicken (breasts, tenders, or thighs), cut into bite-size pieces	1½ cups frozen corn
1 teaspoon dried thyme	1½ cups frozen baby lima beans
1 teaspoon smoked paprika	One 14½-ounce can fire-roasted diced tomatoes and their liquid
1 teaspoon fine sea salt	
½ teaspoon freshly ground black pepper	2 tablespoons tomato paste
1 cup low-sodium chicken	Cornbread, for serving

1. Select the Sauté setting on the Instant Pot and heat the oil and garlic for 2 minutes, until the garlic is bubbling but not browned. Add the onion and sauté for 3 minutes, until it begins to soften. Add the chicken and sauté for 3 minutes more, until mostly opaque. The chicken does not have to be cooked through. Add the thyme, paprika, salt, and pepper and sauté for 1 minute more. 2. Stir in the broth, hot sauce, vinegar, corn, and lima beans. Add the diced tomatoes and their liquid in an even layer and dollop the tomato paste on top. Do not stir them in. 3. Secure the lid and set the Pressure Release to Sealing. Press the Cancel button to reset the cooking program, then select the Pressure Cook or Manual setting and set the cooking time for 5 minutes at high pressure. (The pot will take about 15 minutes to come up to pressure before the cooking program begins.) 4. When the cooking program ends, let the pressure release naturally for at least 10 minutes, then move the Pressure Release to Venting to release any remaining steam. Open the pot and stir the stew to

mix all of the ingredients. 5. Ladle the stew into bowls and serve hot, with cornbread alongside.

Per Serving

Calories: 349 | fat: 7g | protein: 40g | carbs: 17g | sugars: 7g | fiber: 7g | sodium: 535mg

Creamy Chicken Wild Rice Soup

Prep time: 15 minutes | Cook time: 15 minutes | Serves 5

2 tablespoons margarine	Long Grain & Wild Rice Fast Cook
½ cup yellow onion, diced	
¾ cup carrots, diced	2 14-ounce cans low-sodium chicken broth
¾ cup sliced mushrooms (about 3–4 mushrooms)	
	1 cup skim milk
½ pound chicken breast, diced into 1-inch cubes	1 cup evaporated skim milk
	2 ounces fat-free cream cheese
6.2-ounce box Uncle Ben's	2 tablespoons cornstarch

1. Select the Sauté feature and add the margarine, onion, carrots, and mushrooms to the inner pot. Sauté for about 5 minutes until onions are translucent and soft. 2. Add the cubed chicken and seasoning packet from the Uncle Ben's box and stir to combine. 3. Add the rice and chicken broth. Select Manual, high pressure, then lock the lid and make sure the vent is set to sealing. Set the time for 5 minutes. 4. After the cooking time ends, allow it to stay on Keep Warm for 5 minutes and then quick release the pressure. 5. Remove the lid; change the setting to the Sauté function again. 6. Add the skim milk, evaporated milk, and cream cheese. Stir to melt. 7. In a small bowl, mix the cornstarch with a little bit of water to dissolve, then add to the soup to thicken.

Per Serving

Calories: 316 | fat: 7g | protein: 27g | carbs: 35g | sugars: 10g | fiber: 1g | sodium: 638mg

Spicy Turkey Chili

Prep time: 10 minutes | Cook time: 50 minutes | Serves 6

2 onions, chopped	kidney or pinto beans
2 garlic cloves, minced	2 cups canned tomatoes with liquid
½ cup chopped green bell pepper	
	1 cup low-sodium chicken broth
1 tablespoon extra-virgin olive oil	
	2 tablespoon chili powder
1 pound lean ground turkey breast meat	2 teaspoons cumin
	Freshly ground black pepper
2 cups cooked (not canned)	

1. In a large saucepan, sauté the onion, garlic, and green pepper in the oil for 10 minutes. Add the turkey, and sauté until the turkey is cooked, about 5–10 minutes. Drain any fat away. 2. Add the remaining ingredients, bring to a boil, lower the heat, and simmer uncovered for 30 minutes. Add additional chili powder if you like your chili extra spicy.

Per Serving

Calories: 214 | fat: 9.94g | protein: 20.55g | carbs: 11.57g | sugars: 4.11g | fiber: 2.2g | sodium: 363mg

Lentil Soup

Prep time: 10 minutes | Cook time: 55 minutes | Serves 8

1 large onion, diced
1 large carrot, peeled and diced
2 stalks celery, diced
2 tablespoons extra-virgin olive oil
1 pound lentils

1½ quarts low-sodium chicken or beef broth
2 medium russet or white potatoes, peeled and diced
1 tablespoon finely chopped fresh oregano
1 teaspoon finely chopped fresh thyme

1. In a stockpot or Dutch oven, sauté the onion, carrot, and celery in the olive oil for 10 minutes. Add the lentils, broth, and potatoes. 2. Continue to cook for 30–45 minutes, adding the oregano and thyme 15 minutes before serving. Soup will keep for 3 days in the refrigerator or can be frozen for 3 months.

Per Serving

Calories: 174 | fat: 1.63g | protein: 7.71g | carbs: 36.34g | sugars: 1.88g | fiber: 3g | sodium: 81mg

Slow Cooker Chicken and Vegetable Soup

Prep time: 10 minutes | Cook time: 4 hours | Serves 4

1 medium potato, peeled and chopped into 1-inch pieces
3 celery stalks, chopped into 1-inch pieces
2 cups chopped baby carrots
1 cup chopped white onion
2 cups chopped green beans

2 cups low-sodium chicken broth
2 tablespoons tomato paste
2 tablespoons Italian seasoning
1 pound boneless, skinless chicken breasts, chopped
Freshly ground black pepper

1. Put the potato, celery, carrots, onion, green beans, broth, tomato paste, Italian seasoning, and chicken into a slow cooker and cook on high for 4 hours. 2. Season with freshly ground black pepper.

Per Serving

Calories: 256 | fat: 1.84g | protein: 25.68g | carbs: 36.11g | sugars: 7.14g | fiber: 6.8g | sodium: 980mg

West African–Inspired Peanut Soup

Prep time: 10 minutes | Cook time: 20 minutes | Serves 4 to 6

6 garlic cloves, minced
1½-inch piece ginger, grated
1 jalapeño pepper, stemmed, halved, and minced, divided
Kosher salt
2 (14-ounce) cans coconut milk, divided
2 tablespoons vegetable oil, divided
1 teaspoon turmeric

½ cup unsweetened peanut butter
8 cups vegetable broth
2 sweet potatoes, cut into ½-inch cubes
1 bunch collard greens, chopped
Juice of 1 lime
Freshly ground black pepper
½ cup chopped cilantro

1. Place the garlic, ginger, half the jalapeño, and a pinch of salt in a mound on a cutting board. Use the flat of your knife to create a paste. The paste can also be made in a food processor or with a mortar and pestle. 2. Scoop 3 tablespoons of the solid white coconut fat off the top of one can of coconut milk and place it in a large Dutch oven or stockpot. Add 1 tablespoon of vegetable oil to the coconut fat and heat over medium-high heat, stirring frequently, until the coconut fat separates and the solids start to sizzle, about 2 minutes. Continue cooking, stirring constantly, until the solids turn pale golden brown, about 1 minute longer. Add the garlic paste, turmeric, and peanut butter. Cook, stirring, until aromatic, about 30 seconds. 3. Add the remaining coconut milk from both cans, the broth, and sweet potatoes. Bring the soup to a boil, reduce the heat to low, and simmer until the sweet potatoes are tender, about 15 minutes. 4. When the potatoes are cooked through, use a large spoon to smash about half of the sweet potatoes against the side of the stockpot to help thicken the stew. Add the collard greens and lime juice. 5. Season the soup to taste with salt and pepper and serve topped with cilantro and the remaining minced jalapeños. 6. Store the cooled soup in an airtight container in the refrigerator for 3 to 5 days.

Per Serving

Calories: 312 | fat: 11.67g | protein: 10.65g | carbs: 44.52g | sugars: 14.78g | fiber: 9.1g | sodium: 866mg

Appendix 1 Measurement Conversion Chart

MEASUREMENT CONVERSION CHART

VOLUME EQUIVALENTS(DRY)

US STANDARD	METRIC (APPROXIMATE)
1/8 teaspoon	0.5 mL
1/4 teaspoon	1 mL
1/2 teaspoon	2 mL
3/4 teaspoon	4 mL
1 teaspoon	5 mL
1 tablespoon	15 mL
1/4 cup	59 mL
1/2 cup	118 mL
3/4 cup	177 mL
1 cup	235 mL
2 cups	475 mL
3 cups	700 mL
4 cups	1 L

VOLUME EQUIVALENTS(LIQUID)

US STANDARD	US STANDARD (OUNCES)	METRIC (APPROXIMATE)
2 tablespoons	1 fl.oz.	30 mL
1/4 cup	2 fl.oz.	60 mL
1/2 cup	4 fl.oz.	120 mL
1 cup	8 fl.oz.	240 mL
1 1/2 cup	12 fl.oz.	355 mL
2 cups or 1 pint	16 fl.oz.	475 mL
4 cups or 1 quart	32 fl.oz.	1 L
1 gallon	128 fl.oz.	4 L

TEMPERATURES EQUIVALENTS

FAHRENHEIT(F)	CELSIUS(C) (APPROXIMATE)
225 °F	107 °C
250 °F	120 °C
275 °F	135 °C
300 °F	150 °C
325 °F	160 °C
350 °F	180 °C
375 °F	190 °C
400 °F	205 °C
425 °F	220 °C
450 °F	235 °C
475 °F	245 °C
500 °F	260 °C

WEIGHT EQUIVALENTS

US STANDARD	METRIC (APPROXIMATE)
1 ounce	28 g
2 ounces	57 g
5 ounces	142 g
10 ounces	284 g
15 ounces	425 g
16 ounces (1 pound)	455 g
1.5 pounds	680 g
2 pounds	907 g

Appendix 2 The Dirty Dozen and Clean Fifteen

The Dirty Dozen and Clean Fifteen

The Environmental Working Group (EWG) is a nonprofit, nonpartisan organization dedicated to protecting human health and the environment Its mission is to empower people to live healthier lives in a healthier environment. This organization publishes an annual list of the twelve kinds of produce, in sequence, that have the highest amount of pesticide residue-the Dirty Dozen-as well as a list of the fifteen kinds ofproduce that have the least amount of pesticide residue-the Clean Fifteen.

THE DIRTY DOZEN

- The 2016 Dirty Dozen includes the following produce. These are considered among the year's most important produce to buy organic:

Strawberries	Spinach
Apples	Tomatoes
Nectarines	Bell peppers
Peaches	Cherry tomatoes
Celery	Cucumbers
Grapes	Kale/collard greens
Cherries	Hot peppers

- *The Dirty Dozen list contains two additional itemskale/collard greens and hot peppers-because they tend to contain trace levels of highly hazardous pesticides.*

THE CLEAN FIFTEEN

- The least critical to buy organically are the Clean Fifteen list. The following are on the 2016 list:

Avocados	Papayas
Corn	Kiw
Pineapples	Eggplant
Cabbage	Honeydew
Sweet peas	Grapefruit
Onions	Cantaloupe
Asparagus	Cauliflower
Mangos	

- *Some of the sweet corn sold in the United States are made from genetically engineered (GE) seedstock. Buy organic varieties of these crops to avoid GE produce.*

Appendix 3 Recipes Index

A

all-purpose flour
Double-Ginger Cookies	87

almond
Dreamy Caesar Dressing	32
Peach Shortcake	81
Almond Pesto Salmon	64
Wild Rice Salad with Cranberries and Almonds	20

almond flour
Pumpkin Spice Muffins	12
Low-Carb Peanut Butter Pancakes	18
Oatmeal Cookies	83
Cherry Almond Cobbler	81
Grain-Free Parmesan Chicken	59

almond milk
Easy Breakfast Chia Pudding	13
Ranch Vegetable Dip and Dressing	31
Cinnamon Overnight Oats	9
Pumpkin Cheesecake Smoothie	83

almond milkv
No-Added-Sugar Orange and Cream Slushy	86

apple
Apple Crunch	84
Fried Apples	85
Apple-Bulgur Salad	76
Lentil-Apple Salad	78
Dutch Oven Apple Pork Chops	40

applesauce
Grain-Free Applesauce Crêpes	12

artichoke heart
Sautéed Chicken with Artichoke Hearts	52
Baked Oysters	61
Greek Island Potato Salad	77

arugula
Fiber-Full Chicken Tostadas	56

asparagus
Asparagus and Bell Pepper Strata	10
Asparagus with Vinaigrette	21
Chinese Asparagus	21
Roasted Asparagus–Berry Salad	74
Coconut Lime Chicken	54
Creamy Cod with Asparagus	66
Scallops and Asparagus Skillet	67
Roasted Tilapia and Vegetables	63

avocado
Baked Avocado and Egg	10
Rotisserie Chicken and Avocado Salad	75
Crab-Stuffed Avocado Boats	64
Creamy Green Smoothie	13
Salsa Makeover	30

B

banana
Chocolate Baked Bananas	86
Banana Pineapple Freeze	87
Blueberry Coconut Breakfast Cookies	13
Crepe Cakes	18
Mango Nice Cream	85
Peach and Almond Meal Fritters	86

basil
5-Minute Pesto	31

bean sprout
Sherried Peppers with Bean Sprouts	23

beef
Smothered Sirloin	35
Beef Burgundy	35
Asian Steak Salad	35
Salisbury Steaks with Seared Cauliflower	36
Slow Cooker Ropa Vieja	36
Herbed Chipotle Pot Roast	37
Homey Pot Roast	38
Traditional Beef Stroganoff	39
Roasted Beef with Peppercorn Sauce	43
Sloppy Joes	44
Beef Stew	45
Rosemary Roast Beef	45
Butterflied Beef Eye Roast	46
Cheeseburger Wedge Salad	72
Favorite Chili	92
Savory Beef Stew with Mushrooms and Turnips	95
Instantly Good Beef Stew	97
Hearty Beef and Veggie Stew	97
Taco Soup	98

beef chuck
Red Wine Pot Roast with Winter Vegetables	41
Easy Pot Roast and Vegetables	43
Mediterranean Beef Steaks	46

beet
Roasted Beets, Carrots, and Parsnips	20
Quinoa, Beet, and Greens Salad	75
Sweet Beet Grain Bowl	76

bell pepper

Chunky Red Pepper and Tomato Sauce	25
Roasted Red Pepper Spread	31
Asparagus and Bell Pepper Strata	10
Sherried Peppers with Bean Sprouts	23
Orange Chicken Thighs with Bell Peppers	56
Veggie And Egg White Scramble With Pepper Jack Cheese	11
Lentil Salad	71
Italian Wild Mushrooms	28
Pork Mole Quesadillas	37
Italian Sausages with Peppers and Onions	35
Spicy Shrimp Fajitas	62
Steak with Bell Pepper	39
Steak Fajita Bake	44
Spinach and Sweet Pepper Poppers	22

berry

Mixed-Berry Snack Cake	82

black bean

Black Bean Breakfast Burrito	17
Tortilla-Bean Salad	72
Chipotle Black Bean Brownies	88
Catfish with Corn and Pepper Relish	69
Black Bean, Turmeric, and Cauliflower Tortilla Soup	94
Jerk Chicken Casserole	51
Cauli-Curry Bean Soup	92
Coddled Huevos Rancheros	11
Southwestern Bean Soup with Corn Dumplings	96
Four-Bean Field Stew	93
Peanut Butter Fudge Brownies	83
Rainbow Quinoa Salad	73
Calypso Shrimp with Black Bean Salsa	68

blackberry

Ginger Blackberry Bliss Smoothie Bowl	13
Blueberry-Chia Smoothie	10
Berry–French Toast Stratas	10
Blueberry Chocolate Clusters	88
Baked Berry Cups with Crispy Cinnamon Wedges	88
Goji Berry Muesli	17
Blueberry Cornmeal Muffins	9
Mixed-Berry Cream Tart	82
Creamy Blueberry Quesadillas	13

bread

Simple Bread Pudding	87
Crumb Pie Shell	88
Toads In Holes	11
French Onion Soup	93
Sweet Potato Toasts	13

broccoli

Broccoli Cauliflower Bake	21
Garlic Roasted Broccoli	23
Sautéed Lemon Broccoli and Kale	23
Sautéed Mixed Vegetables	25
Ginger Broccoli	27
Broccoli Slaw Crab Salad	75
Teriyaki Chicken and Broccoli	48

Pork Tenderloin Stir-Fry	45
Ginger-Glazed Salmon and Broccoli	68
Lemon Pepper Tilapia with Broccoli and Carrots	65
Turkey Divan Casserole	54

brown rice

Crab and Rice Salad	74
Greek Rice Salad	74
Greek Chicken Stuffed Peppers	51
Asian Mushroom-Chicken Soup	57
Asian Salmon in a Packet	61

Brussels sprout

Lemony Brussels Sprouts with Poppy Seeds	22
Brussels Sprouts with Pecans and Gorgonzola	24
Sun-Dried Tomato Brussels Sprouts	26
Shaved Brussels Sprouts and Kale with Poppy Seed Dressing	75
Beef Stew	45
One-Pan Chicken Dinner	48
Chicken Tender and Brussels Sprout Cobb Salad	73

buckwheat flour

Easy Buckwheat Crêpes	17

bulgur

Apple-Bulgur Salad	76

buttermilk

Ranch Dressing	32

butternut squash

Butternut Squash Soup	95
Cauliflower and Butternut Squash Mac and Cheese	28
Pumpkin Soup	93
Turkey–Butternut Squash Ragout	50

C

cabbage

Charred Miso Cabbage	24
Dijon Roast Cabbage	25
Sweet-and-Sour Cabbage Slaw	27
Cheesy Stuffed Cabbage	54
Make-Ahead Apple, Carrot, and Cabbage Slaw	74
Cabbage Slaw Salad	76
Power Salad	77
Hearty Italian Minestrone	93
Sloppy Joes	44
Garlicky Cabbage and Collard Greens	25
Turkey Cabbage Soup	49

carrot

Vegetable Medley	24
Carrots Marsala	27
Vegetable broth	30
Roasted Carrot and Quinoa with Goat Cheese	73
Zucchini, Carrot, and Fennel Salad	79
Carrot Soup	94
Thai Peanut, Carrot, and Shrimp Soup	94
Slow Cooker Chicken and Vegetable Soup	99
Hearty Beef and Veggie Stew	97

Roasted Beets, Carrots, and Parsnips	20
Sweet-and-Sour Cabbage Slaw	27
Make-Ahead Apple, Carrot, and Cabbage Slaw	74
Cabbage Slaw Salad	76
Thai Yellow Curry with Chicken Meatballs	49
Wine-Poached Chicken with Herbs and Vegetables	52
Shredded Buffalo Chicken	52
Chicken Noodle Soup	91
Chock-Full-of-Vegetables Chicken Soup	90
Potlikker Soup	96
African Peanut Stew	94

cashew

Strawberry Cheesecake in a Jar	85

catfish

Catfish with Corn and Pepper Relish	69

cauliflower

Cauliflower Scramble	18
Cauliflower "Mashed Potatoes"	22
Parmesan Cauliflower Mash	24
Horseradish Mashed Cauliflower	26
Cheesy Cauli Bake	28
Cauliflower and Butternut Squash Mac and Cheese	28
Spicy Roasted Cauliflower with Lime	28
Ranch Vegetable Dip and Dressing	31
Pomegranate "Tabbouleh" with Cauliflower	71
Black Bean, Turmeric, and Cauliflower Tortilla Soup	94
Cauliflower Chili	97
Slow Cooker Ropa Vieja	36
Broccoli Cauliflower Bake	21
Sautéed Mixed Vegetables	25
Lean Green Avocado Mashed Potatoes	20
Sunflower-Tuna-Cauliflower Salad	77

celery

Ham and Potato Chowder	92

cheese

Dulce de Leche Fillo Cups	83
Crustless Key Lime Cheesecake	86
Low-Fat Cream Cheese Frosting	87
Gouda Egg Casserole	14
Egg Bites with Sausage and Peppers	18
Two-Cheese Grits	9
Goat Cheese–Stuffed Pears	83
Breakfast Meatballs	17
Shredded Potato Omelet	14

cherry

Cherry Almond Cobbler	81
Lamb Chops with Cherry Glaze	44

cherry tomato

Tantalizing Jerked Chicken	59
Mediterranean-Style Cod	63

chia seed

Easy Breakfast Chia Pudding	13

chicken

Italian Turkey Sausage Meatballs	30

Thai Yellow Curry with Chicken Meatballs	49
Wine-Poached Chicken with Herbs and Vegetables	52
Nutty Deconstructed Salad	72
Rotisserie Chicken and Avocado Salad	75
Chinese Chicken Salad	77
Chicken Brunswick Stew	98

chicken breast

Teriyaki Chicken and Broccoli	48
One-Pan Chicken Dinner	48
Coconut Chicken Curry	50
Greek Chicken Stuffed Peppers	51
Chicken with Mushroom Cream Sauce	51
Sautéed Chicken with Artichoke Hearts	52
Shredded Buffalo Chicken	52
Peppered Chicken with Balsamic Kale	52
Baked Chicken Stuffed with Collard Greens	53
Coconut Lime Chicken	54
Chicken with Lemon Caper Pan Sauce	55
Saffron-Spiced Chicken Breasts	55
Ginger Curry Chicken Kabobs	56
Fiber-Full Chicken Tostadas	56
Asian Mushroom-Chicken Soup	57
Fajita-Stuffed Chicken Breast	57
Cast Iron Hot Chicken	57
Chicken Paprika	58
Orange Chicken	58
Chicken in Wine	58
Tantalizing Jerked Chicken	59
Grain-Free Parmesan Chicken	59
Curried Chicken Salad	73
Chicken Noodle Soup	91
Comforting Chicken and Mushroom Soup	93
Creamy Chicken Wild Rice Soup	98

chicken leg quarter

Smoky Chicken Leg Quarters	56

chicken tender

Chicken Tender and Brussels Sprout Cobb Salad	73
Chock-Full-of-Vegetables Chicken Soup	90

chicken thigh

Cilantro Lime Chicken Thighs	48
Chicken Patties	49
Tangy Barbecue Strawberry-Peach Chicken	50
Jerk Chicken Casserole	51
Lemony Chicken Thighs	53
Italian Chicken Thighs	54
Orange Chicken Thighs with Bell Peppers	56
Speedy Chicken Cacciatore	57
Ginger Turmeric Chicken Thighs	58
Jerk Chicken Thighs	58

chickpea

Teriyaki Chickpeas	27
Green Chickpea Hummus	31
Mediterranean Chef Salad	74
Chickpea Salad	76
Three Bean and Basil Salad	78
Chickpea "Tuna" Salad	78

Freshened-Up French Onion Soup 90
Cauli-Curry Bean Soup 92
Roasted Red Pepper Spread 31

chocolate
Chocolate Almond Butter Fudge 81
Chipotle Black Bean Brownies 88
Blueberry Chocolate Clusters 88

coconut flour
Grain-Free Applesauce Crêpes 12

coconut milk
Coffee and Cream Pops 86
Chocolate Almond Butter Fudge 81
West African–Inspired Peanut Soup 99

cod
Mediterranean-Style Cod 63
Creamy Cod with Asparagus 66
Crispy Fish Sticks 66
Friday Night Fish Fry 66

collard greens
Garlicky Cabbage and Collard Greens 25
Pumpkin Soup 93
Potlikker Soup 96
Baked Chicken Stuffed with Collard Greens 53

corn
Taco Soup 98
Chicken Brunswick Stew 98
Mexican Tortilla Soup 97

corn grits
Savory Grits 16

cornmeal
Hoe Cakes 15

couscous
Mediterranean Salmon with Whole-Wheat Couscous 63

crab
Crab-Stuffed Avocado Boats 64

crab meat
Broccoli Slaw Crab Salad 75
Crab and Rice Salad 74

cranberry
Chocolate Chip and Cranberry Cookies 87

cucumber
Greek Rice Salad 74
Chickpea "Tuna" Salad 78
Lamb Kofta Meatballs with Cucumber Quick-Pickled Salad 44
Garden-Fresh Greek Salad 71

D

delicata squash
Roasted Delicata Squash 21

E

edamame
Power Salad 77
Chickpea Salad 76
Edamame and Walnut Salad 79

egg
Toads In Holes 11
Coddled Huevos Rancheros 11
Veggie And Egg White Scramble With Pepper Jack Cheese 11
Blueberry Coconut Breakfast Cookies 13
Gouda Egg Casserole 14
Cinnamon French Toast 15
Breakfast Casserole 15
Crepe Cakes 18
Egg Bites with Sausage and Peppers 18
Egg Drop Soup 96
Pumpkin Spice Muffins 12
Low-Carb Peanut Butter Pancakes 18
Baked Avocado and Egg 10
Berry–French Toast Stratas 10
Crustless Key Lime Cheesecake 86
Pumpkin–Peanut Butter Single-Serve Muffins 14
Spinach and Feta Egg Bake 9
Easy Sweet Potato and Egg Sandwiches 14
Whole-Grain Strawberry Pancakes 12
Pumpkin Apple Waffles 17

eggplant
Ratatouille Baked Eggs 11

F

farro
Sweet Beet Grain Bowl 76

flank steak
Mediterranean Steak Sandwiches 37
Steak Gyro Platter 40
Spinach and Provolone Steak Rolls 42

flounder
Air Fryer Fish Fry 66

flour
Basic Pie Crust 81

G

grape
Nutty Deconstructed Salad 72
green bean
Green Beans with Garlic and Onion 22
Nutmeg Green Beans 25
Green Beans with Red Peppers 26
Green Ginger Soup 90
Slow Cooker Chicken and Vegetable Soup 99
Roasted Halibut with Red Peppers, Green Beans, and Onions 64
Romaine Lettuce Salad with Cranberry, Feta, and Beans 76
Salmon en Papillote 65

| 105

Salmon Niçoise Salad 72

grits
Two-Cheese Grits 9

H

halibut
Roasted Halibut with Red Peppers, Green Beans, and Onions 64
Halibut with Lime and Cilantro 67

ham hock
French Market Soup 95

K

kale
Creamy Green Smoothie 13
Wilted Kale and Chard 23
African Peanut Stew 94
Tomato and Kale Soup 95
Black Bean Breakfast Burrito 17
Sautéed Lemon Broccoli and Kale 23
Shaved Brussels Sprouts and Kale with Poppy Seed Dressing 75
Peppered Chicken with Balsamic Kale 52
Coconut, Miso, and Sweet Potato White Bean Chili 91

kidney bean
Southwestern Bean Soup with Corn Dumplings 96
Three Bean and Basil Salad 78

L

lamb
Slow-Cooked Simple Lamb and Vegetable Stew 42
Herb-Crusted Lamb Chops 43
Lamb Kofta Meatballs with Cucumber Quick-Pickled Salad 44
Lamb Chops with Cherry Glaze 44

lamb shoulder
Spiced Lamb Stew 41

lentil
Lentil, Squash, and Tomato Omelet 9
Lentil Salad 71
Lentil-Apple Salad 78
Lentil Soup 99

lettuce
Garden-Fresh Greek Salad 71
Romaine Lettuce Salad with Cranberry, Feta, and Beans 76
Grilled Romaine with White Beans 77
Grilled Hearts of Romaine with Buttermilk Dressing 78
Asian Steak Salad 35
Curried Chicken Salad 73
Mediterranean Steak Sandwiches 37
Steak Gyro Platter 40

lima bean
Four-Bean Field Stew 93

lobster
Lobster Fricassee 69

M

mandarin orange
Mandarin Orange–Millet Breakfast Bowl 16

mango
Mango Nice Cream 85
Mango-Glazed Pork Tenderloin Roast 39
Shrimp Burgers with Fruity Salsa and Salad 65

milk
Low-Calorie, Fat-Free Whipped Cream 85
Simple Bread Pudding 87
Easy Buckwheat Crêpes 17
Savory Grits 16
Cinnamon French Toast 15

millet
Mandarin Orange–Millet Breakfast Bowl 16

mushroom
Italian Wild Mushrooms 28
Beef Burgundy 35
Salisbury Steaks with Seared Cauliflower 36
Herbed Chipotle Pot Roast 37
Savory Beef Stew with Mushrooms and Turnips 95
Chicken with Mushroom Cream Sauce 51
Chicken Paprika 58
Comforting Chicken and Mushroom Soup 93
Creamy Chicken Wild Rice Soup 98
Lobster Fricassee 69
Garlic Beef Stroganoff 38
Italian Beef Kebabs 42
Beef and Vegetable Shish Kabobs 44
Tofu, Kale, and Mushroom Breakfast Scramble 12
Tasty Tomato Soup 90
Mushroom-Sage Stuffed Turkey Breast 50

mussel
Seafood Stew 68

N

navy bean
Pico de Gallo Navy Beans 24
Coconut, Miso, and Sweet Potato White Bean Chili 91

nut
Toasted Nuts 32

O

oat
Cinnamon Overnight Oats 9
Goji Berry Muesli 17
5-Ingredient Chunky Cherry and Peanut Butter Cookies 82
Peanut Butter Fudge Brownies 83

Oatmeal Cookies 83
Oatmeal Chippers 85
Quick Yummy Peaches 84
Sweet Potato Breakfast Bites 16
Chewy Chocolate-Oat Bars 84

oat flour
Blueberry Cornmeal Muffins 9
Oatmeal Chippers 85

onion
Caramelized Onions 22
French Onion Soup 93
Smothered Sirloin 35
Ginger Broccoli 27
Vegetable broth 30
Freshened-Up French Onion Soup 90
Breakfast Hash 15
Basic Marinara 32

orange
Orange Dijon Dressing 33
No-Added-Sugar Orange and Cream Slushy 86

oyster
Baked Oysters 61

P

parsnip
Red Wine Pot Roast with Winter Vegetables 41
Vegetable Medley 24

pea
Herbed Spring Peas 71

peach
Peach Shortcake 81
Quick Yummy Peaches 84
Grilled Peach and Coconut Yogurt Bowls 84
Peach and Almond Meal Fritters 86
Tangy Barbecue Strawberry-Peach Chicken 50
First-of-the-Season Tomato, Peach, and Strawberry Salad 78

peanut butter
5-Ingredient Chunky Cherry and Peanut Butter Cookies 82

pear
Goat Cheese–Stuffed Pears 83

pecan
Brussels Sprouts with Pecans and Gorgonzola 24
Tilapia with Pecans 67

pine nut
5-Minute Pesto 31

pineapple
Creamy Pineapple-Pecan Dessert Squares 82
Broiled Pineapple 84
Banana Pineapple Freeze 87

pinto bean
Cauliflower Chili 97
Slow-Cooked Pork Burrito Bowls 43
Turkey and Pinto Chili 91
Spicy Turkey Chili 98

plum tomato
First-of-the-Season Tomato, Peach, and Strawberry Salad 78

pollock
Blackened Pollock 66

pork
Breakfast Meatballs 17
Pork Butt Roast 45

pork chop
Pork Mole Quesadillas 37
Dutch Oven Apple Pork Chops 40
Sage-Parmesan Pork Chops 41

pork shoulder
Open-Faced Pulled Pork 40
Slow-Cooked Pork Burrito Bowls 43

pork tenderloin
Mustard Herb Pork Tenderloin 38
Mango-Glazed Pork Tenderloin Roast 39
Pork Tenderloin Stir-Fry 45

potato
Golden Potato Cakes 10
Shredded Potato Omelet 14
Breakfast Hash 15
Hash Browns 15
Lean Green Avocado Mashed Potatoes 20
Ham and Potato Chowder 92
Dreamy Caesar Dressing 32
Homey Pot Roast 38
Instantly Good Beef Stew 97
Easy Pot Roast and Vegetables 43
Lentil Soup 99

pumpkin
Pumpkin–Peanut Butter Single-Serve Muffins 14
Pumpkin Cheesecake Smoothie 83

quinoa
Moreish Lemony Quinoa 23
Rainbow Quinoa Salad 73
Quinoa, Beet, and Greens Salad 75
Roasted Carrot and Quinoa with Goat Cheese 73
Unstuffed Peppers with Ground Turkey and Quinoa 48
Turkey and Quinoa Caprese Casserole 51

R

radish
Parmesan-Rosemary Radishes 21
Garlic Herb Radishes 27
Garlic Roasted Radishes 27

| 107

raspberry
Baked Berry Cups with Crispy Cinnamon Wedges	88

red potato
Potatoes with Parsley	26
Italian Potato Salad	71
Greek Island Potato Salad	77

round steak
Zesty Swiss Steak	37
Garlic Beef Stroganoff	38
Creole Steak	42

S

salmon
Asian Salmon in a Packet	61
Roasted Salmon with Honey-Mustard Sauce	61
Teriyaki Salmon	62
Mediterranean Salmon with Whole-Wheat Couscous	63
Almond Pesto Salmon	64
Salmon en Papillote	65
Salmon Florentine	67
Ginger-Glazed Salmon and Broccoli	68
Citrus-Glazed Salmon	68
Grilled Salmon with Dill Sauce	69
Salmon Niçoise Salad	72

salsa
Salsa Makeover	30

sausage
Italian Sausages with Peppers and Onions	35

scallops
Scallops and Asparagus Skillet	67

short rib
Short Ribs with Chimichurri	40

shrimp
Quick Shrimp Skewers	62
Shrimp with Tomatoes and Feta	62
Spicy Shrimp Fajitas	62
Savory Shrimp	63
Shrimp Burgers with Fruity Salsa and Salad	65
Greek Scampi	67
Calypso Shrimp with Black Bean Salsa	68
Baked Garlic Scampi	69
Thai Peanut, Carrot, and Shrimp Soup	94
Seafood Stew	68

sirloin steak
Grilled Steak and Vegetables	36
Quick Steak Tacos	38
Steak with Bell Pepper	39
Italian Beef Kebabs	42
Steak Fajita Bake	44
Beef and Vegetable Shish Kabobs	44

sole
Spicy Citrus Sole	61
Broiled Sole with Mustard Sauce	62

soy milk
Blueberry-Chia Smoothie	10

spinach
Spinach and Feta Egg Bake	9
Spinach and Sweet Pepper Poppers	22
Strawberry-Spinach Salad	75
Edamame and Walnut Salad	79
Asparagus with Vinaigrette	21
Ginger Blackberry Bliss Smoothie Bowl	13
Mediterranean Chef Salad	74
Spinach and Provolone Steak Rolls	42
Blackened Pollock	66
Salmon Florentine	67

strawberry
Strawberry Chia Pudding	81
Mixed-Berry Cream Tart	82
Strawberry Cheesecake in a Jar	85
Roasted Asparagus–Berry Salad	74
Dulce de Leche Fillo Cups	83
Strawberry-Spinach Salad	75

sweet potato
Sweet Potato Toasts	13
Easy Sweet Potato and Egg Sandwiches	14
Sweet Potato Breakfast Bites	16
Chipotle Twice-Baked Sweet Potatoes	20
Taco Stuffed Sweet Potatoes	49
Roasted Tomato and Sweet Potato Soup	96
West African–Inspired Peanut Soup	99
Coconut Chicken Curry	50
Spiced Lamb Stew	41
Herb-Roasted Turkey and Vegetables	55

Swiss chard
Wilted Kale and Chard	23

swordfish
Grilled Rosemary Swordfish	64

tenderloin steak
Tenderloin with Crispy Shallots	39

T

tilapia
Roasted Tilapia and Vegetables	63
Chili Tilapia	64
Lemon Pepper Tilapia with Broccoli and Carrots	65
Tilapia with Pecans	67

tofu
Tofu, Kale, and Mushroom Breakfast Scramble	12
Soft-Baked Tamari Tofu	23
Cauliflower Scramble	18

tomato
Spicy Tomato Smoothie	12
Basic Marinara	32
Low-Sodium Salsa	33
Tasty Tomato Soup	90

French Market Soup	95
Cheeseburger Wedge Salad	72
Favorite Chili	92
Tortilla-Bean Salad	72
Pomegranate "Tabbouleh" with Cauliflower	71
Green Beans with Red Peppers	26
Tomato and Kale Soup	95
Pico de Gallo Navy Beans	24
Creole Steak	42
Shrimp with Tomatoes and Feta	62
Greek Scampi	67
Grilled Steak and Vegetables	36
Quick Steak Tacos	38
Roasted Tomato and Sweet Potato Soup	96
Tomato Tuna Melts	69
Unstuffed Cabbage Soup	92
Zucchini on the Half Shell	26

tomato juice

Spicy Tomato Smoothie	12

tortilla

Creamy Blueberry Quesadillas	13

tuna

Tuna Steak	64
Tomato Tuna Melts	69
Sunflower-Tuna-Cauliflower Salad	77

turkey

Unstuffed Peppers with Ground Turkey and Quinoa	48
Turkey Cabbage Soup	49
Turkey and Quinoa Caprese Casserole	51
Teriyaki Turkey Meatballs	53
Wild Rice and Turkey Casserole	53
Turkey Divan Casserole	54
Turkey and Pinto Chili	91
Unstuffed Cabbage Soup	92
Cheesy Stuffed Cabbage	54
Taco Stuffed Sweet Potatoes	49

turkey breast

Mushroom-Sage Stuffed Turkey Breast	50
Thanksgiving Turkey Breast	55
Herb-Roasted Turkey and Vegetables	55
Herbed Whole Turkey Breast	59
Spicy Turkey Chili	98

turkey thigh

Turkey–Butternut Squash Ragout	50

turnip

Slow-Cooked Simple Lamb and Vegetable Stew	42

W

walnut

Chocolate Chip and Cranberry Cookies	87

water chestnut

Chinese Chicken Salad	77

wheat bran

Bran Apple Muffins	16

white bean

Irresistible White Bean Dip	32
Green Chickpea Hummus	31
Grilled Romaine with White Beans	77

whole wheat flour

Whole-Grain Strawberry Pancakes	12
Bran Apple Muffins	16
Pumpkin Apple Waffles	17
Mixed-Berry Snack Cake	82
Chewy Chocolate-Oat Bars	84

wild rice

Wild Rice Salad with Cranberries and Almonds	20

Y

yogurt

Ranch Dressing	32
Low-Fat Cream Cheese Frosting	87
Grilled Salmon with Dill Sauce	69

Z

zucchini

Ratatouille Baked Eggs	11
Zucchini on the Half Shell	26
Mexican Tortilla Soup	97
Hearty Italian Minestrone	93
Zucchini, Carrot, and Fennel Salad	79
Breakfast Casserole	15
Green Ginger Soup	90
Lentil, Squash, and Tomato Omelet	9